LOVE MORE, BINGE LESS AND STAY FIT

PERMANENT WEIGHT LOSS, USING YOUR MIND INSTEAD OF BEATING UP ON YOUR BODY

ANNIE STERN, BS, NC

authorHOUSE®

AuthorHouse™ LLC
1663 Liberty Drive
Bloomington, IN 47403
www.authorhouse.com
Phone: 1-800-839-8640

Published by AuthorHouse   09/03/2014

ISBN: 978-1-4969-3690-5 (sc)
ISBN: 978-1-4969-3691-2 (hc)
ISBN: 978-1-4969-3689-9 (e)

Contents

Acknowledgments

First and foremost, I give gratitude to my mom. Your love and support are constantly with me. To my dad for raising me with the words, "Hard work always pays off." And to my sister, Szilvi, for believing in me to do this.

I am so grateful to my friends for being there when I needed you: Wenchi Liao, Titanilla Béli, Emily Day, Agnes Berényi, Angela Dayberry and Kity Krebsz.

Frank Wainwright, your encouragement is my strength. You made writing this book feel like a return to myself. For this, I will be forever grateful for you.

Thanks to all of my great nutrition instructors at Bauman College, especially Laura Knoff, for making nutrition more interesting and eye opening. I truly enjoyed your classes.

I couldn't be where I am today without all the great mentors, I've had along the way, especially those of you who inspired me to write this book: Dr. Brené Brown, Gabrielle Bernstein, Marie Forleo, Geneen Roth, Stefanie Nielsen, Jena La Flamme, Teal Swan and Karla McLaren. You are all giants in my life.

Thank you.

This book is about making good decisions by yourself, for yourself.

Annie Stern
San Francisco
2014

Part I
Introduction

The constant struggle to look good and the desire to get thin is obsessive among women and girls, as we think that our happiness is at stake. We want to be valued and loved, and our appearance is often a big part of our identity.

I wrote this book because the mainstream idea behind how to lose weight permanently is so misunderstood—hence the millions of women of all ages around the world who struggle to manage their weight. I want to give away the knowledge I have to anyone who can relate to this issue.

I am a certified holistic nutritionist who was taught that the model of health relies not only on nutrition and physical activity but also on mental attitude, family, work, and community relationships. When it comes to weight management, we need to address behavioral and emotional issues as well as nutritional and metabolic issues. I was excited when I learned there might be much more to the story of weight management than nutrition and exercise.

Although I was looking for answers about weight management during my studies, the question I had in mind became how to keep weight off forever. That is, how can we stop ourselves from losing and gaining the same ten, twenty, thirty, or more pounds over and over again? Jumping on and off diets to lose weight means living in a state of constant pushes and limitations. It doesn't feel good. So, you will fall off the wagon and start gaining the weight again.

If anybody follows the mainstream advice on weight management, he or she will think about nutrition and exercise as the magic bullet. But what if our struggles to keep the weight off with these methods are just one piece of the pie? What if there is much more to the story?

There is no doubt that dieting can make you physically starve for nutrients, and then you binge or overeat, hence the ongoing weight struggle. But what if binging or overeating can happen because of emotional hunger? What if a world exists behind all of your thoughts, beliefs, and feelings that makes you want to eat even if you are not hungry?

Binge eating or overeating are both compulsive eating behaviors. The difference between them is that although, they are both the result of an emotional response, binge eating happens in secrecy, overeating happens around people or in secrecy. Binge eating can include small or large amounts of food. Overeating includes eating to a point where fullness becomes uncomfortable.

Furthermore, what if there are unseen worlds behind your yo-yo dieting patterns, your craziness around food, and body image issues that are the real problems in your weight struggle? Consider the idea that your eating habits might have nothing to do with whether you are hungry, and food consumption could be a self-soothing mechanism you've created. What if I told you that until you find peace with your body or your life, you will never able to manage your weight? Until you understand who you are in your emotions, not only will you never experience permanent weight loss and body happiness but also you will never be truly happy.

Regardless of whether your eating patterns are physically or emotionally driven, until you look behind all the triggers that created the effect, your weight struggle, you will not have enough confidence in your body. Perhaps you gained weight and you want to lose it, or you are thin now and you're worried about gaining weight. Whatever your physical situation is, the guilt and shame around your body will always be there if you don't deal with the emotional aspect.

It took two decades of constant weight struggles, body hate, and craziness around food before I tried to find answers somewhere other than nutrition and exercise. Only then did I slowly understand the reason behind my struggle with my weight.

We often accept things for their appearance and don't want to look behind the curtain. Society has developed an industry worth twenty billion dollars in which people are told to go on diets to lose weight. The beauty industry constantly tells people they are not good enough, so it can sell more products to fix us.

Whenever women suddenly feel fat, it is not an emotion but a byproduct of living in modern society. They constantly absorb the media messages about how to look and what to achieve in life, and when the two don't match up, women take it out on their bodies, as they feel uncertain, scared, or not good enough.

When our social and cultural environments constantly tell us who we are and what our life mission should be, we easily lose touch with ourselves. And then we take action to push down the emotions we don't want to feel. We eat even if we are not hungry. Zoning out or numbing ourselves from our life becomes normal.

It is time to take back your personal power. If you are someone who feels food is your best friend and your worst enemy—if you think your true happiness depends on how you look and if you don't know why you eat when you are not even hungry—this book will give you the answers. More than that, it will help you experience confidence with your body and allow you to step back into your own power.

Additionally, this book will help you to know how to lose weight permanently without gaining and losing pounds all the time. You will find out how to stop being crazy around food and even socialize where food is readily available without going overboard. Understand how you can have your favorite food and still manage your weight as well as how to eat anything but never be triggered to overeat. Eventually, you will discover how to love yourself thin and stay fit. You will learn why self-confidence leads to permanent weight loss and not the other way around. This is a book of self-discovery while learning the meaning of anything that has to do with nutrition, exercise, emotions, mind-set, stable body weight, body image, and happiness.

It is time to create a life that you deserve by getting off the diet-binge cycle created by your restrictive dieting patterns. The time has come for you to release emotional hunger and to overcome your body shame and body image insecurity. My wish is for you to stay fit. I don't want you to avoid changing your body if it is overweight or obese. However, I want you to drop shame, hate, and guilt-ridden behaviors around your body, because you can't really take good care of something you hate. I can only help you release all the triggers that make your body want to hang on to physically driven overeating, binging patterns, or any compulsive behaviors around food if you start from this point. Disliking your body, whatever size it is, only leads to robbing yourself of the option of feeling good about yourself.

Food addictions and eating disorders label women and girls as being sick or flawed. My approach gives you freedom from these labels and helps you to see your struggle for what it is without the guilt and shame. Let's say there is no wagon to fall off of, only lessons so that you can relearn who you are, what makes you happy, and how to live in a world where social and cultural expectations like to put people in a box.

Your soul is an ever-expanding eternity that knows no boundaries, and remembering its identity will lead you to emotional, mental, physical, and spiritual happiness. Your body will find its natural healthy size, so a constant weight struggle will no longer be an issue for you.

Love More, Binge Less, and Stay Fit will lead you toward areas of your life you thought you'd forgotten but still have a vast impact on you. This is the key to mastering your weight struggle.

This is a transformational book. It aims to give you a shift in perception. When you get that change, your excess weight will fall off without effort. I recommend that you take your time reading this book. It is meant to be thought provoking and eye opening.

Although I wrote this specifically for people who struggle with extra weight, someone in the category of anorexia (is underweight, has intense fear of weight gain, eats only small amounts of a few foods) or bulimia (uses diet pills or laxatives, has chronic unhappiness with body size and shape, fears gaining weight and for this reason frequently goes to the bathroom after eating to throw up) can greatly benefit from this information.

I share my own journey of going from someone who based her self-worth on body shape and weight to becoming the best version of herself. I also share stories and experiences from working in this field.

When the idea of writing this book hit me, at first I was reluctant because I didn't want to write about standard weight loss. That's not who I am or what I stand for in my work. This book goes against nutrition and exercise as the ultimate solution for permanent weight loss, and it goes deeper than that. I wanted to write a book that resolves the drama you have around weight, body image, negative self-talk, and food, making it feel like you are in food jail. I wish you to feel free from all of these issues; only then can you become the best version of yourself.

I feel extremely honored to share this process with you, and I hope that while you read this book, you will have the courage to look within yourself. I also hope that you will have the same compassion toward yourself as you would toward your best friend. Be willing to do the work it takes to get to the other side: a life that contains freedom around food, freedom from weight struggles, freedom from body image insecurities, and freedom from the struggle of feeling not good enough. You are enough, right now—perhaps you just don't know it yet.

Part II
The Triggers of All Problems

During the time I wrote the majority of this book, I was also preparing for a big jump: relocating from New York to San Francisco. I stayed in a beautiful cottage for a couple of months, far from the noises, in the countryside of Hungary, where I was born and raised. As I flipped through the responses I got from the questionnaire I gave to hundreds of health club members while I was a fitness manager in Manhattan, the reasons most people have ongoing weight struggles while they are chronic yo-yo dieters became clear.

The Top 4 Reasons

You Have Constant Weight Struggles

▸ Diet Mentality

▸ Live By The "Eat Less, Exercise More" Model

▸ Emotional Appetite

▸ Trapped In Body Image Insecurity And Body Shame

The Triggers of All Problems
Reason #1: Diet Mentality

The standard concept of dieting is based on restricting yourself from specific foods. Whether you call it controlling or limiting your food intake, this falls in the category of a diet mind-set. In the cycle of dieting, most likely you lose weight and then somehow regain it. You may then see yourself as failure. Even though diets never deliver permanent weight loss, you still see the idea of dieting as something good, and you think your ineffective efforts are what caused you to fail. So, you promise to yourself that next time, you will do it differently— you will be better. Once you have a diet mentality, the on-and-off pattern is inevitable and hard to break. Whether you are dieting right now or not, even if you want to give it up, it is difficult. A chronic diet mentality creates destructive weight-loss behaviors, generates anxiety around food and body, and builds weight preoccupation. Although you understand from experience that yo-yo gain and loss comes from dieting, you hope to find the "right" diet that works the next time.

With the help of diet mentality, you pick up beliefs and habits about food to control your body size. For this reason, you might practice any of the following behaviors:

- Constantly thinking about what you ate and what you will eat next; you might check in with yourself regularly to see if you are doing the right things to reshape your body
- Regularly measuring food by counting calories, avoiding certain food groups, and counting grams of fat, carbs, or protein
- Avoiding social gatherings to keep from eating "bad" foods
- Ignoring your body's signs when it becomes hungry and sitting on your hands to not eat
- Using distractions such as drinking more or eating liquid-like foods
- Skipping meals when you feel fat
- Feeling guilty, ashamed, and bad when you eat something you are not supposed to consume

- Building boundaries around food and letting rules dictate your relationship with food
- Thinking about your body weight, size, and shape excessively and weighing yourself multiple times a day; checking yourself in the mirror to judge yourself or being overly concerned what others think about your body
- Engaging in activities to distract yourself from eating; this can take the form of smoking cigarettes, using diet pills, or drinking caffeinated beverages to reduce cravings
- Engaging in an otherwise healthy behavior by compulsively using exercise as a magic pill to shed extra pounds

Three Universal Diet Types

There are three universal types of diets that women and girls start and stop from the moment they become conscious about their body image and want to change its size or shape to get rid of their insecurity. While you are reading the section, check with yourself to see which type of dieter you are.

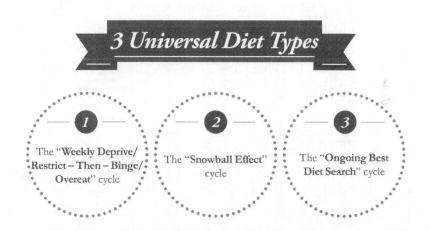

9

The Weekly Deprive-Restrict and Then Binge-Overeat

This cycle usually starts on Monday, and you are pretty well behaved with your diet up until Thursday or Friday. When the weekend comes, for so many different reasons, you slip and you overeat, basically getting off your diet. And then you start a new cycle on Monday with the perfect diet in mind, only to realize as that weekend comes, you are really bored, and you tell yourself you need some real food to spice up your life. With this type of dieting, you most likely go back and forth between restrictive eating and overeating. You might switch between the two over the course of weeks or months or even in one day or a meal. You start with honest, good intentions but somehow we lose control.

The Snowball-Effect

Your weight yo-yos because the motivation behind your diet yo-yos. It is seasonal, and it depends on what's happening in your life. You might have an emergency, a special event, a fitness competition, a crisis, or an important event, or summertime coming up. The bottom line is that losing weight suddenly seems really important for you, so you jump on a diet plan for weeks or months until you pass that special circumstance. The motivation for weight loss is then gone, so you start eating what you are "not supposed to" again as a result of the deprivation you experienced.

The Ongoing Search for the Best Diet

You never really see the permanent results in losing or managing your weight, and you are always looking for the new best diet to give you the ultimate plan. You jump on different diets, mostly those that pop up out in the mainstream, and they promise what you want: easy, fast, and permanent weight loss. But then you realize that these diets take up so much of your willpower that even if they work, you can't sustain them in the long run.

If diets worked, we would all be permanently thin. You demonstrate the diet mentality when you tend to choose off-the-shelf diets that some experts recommend, and you believe you found the magic bullet. As you try to fit your life within these diets, you quit them at some point, even though a lot of them do work. The problem with this type of dieting is that you are either in control or out of control with food. A dieting mind-set pushes you to overeat, binge, or eat compulsively because you will eventually always crave what you can't have. Diets create deprivation symptoms, as you forbid yourself from certain foods or food groups for a while. However, because deprivation is unsustainable, you will eat food that you've forbidden yourself from consuming sooner or later.

Most of us understand intellectually why dieting leads to crash diets, but we still do it because we don't know a better way. Dieting leads to losing weight and getting the body you want sooner than later, no doubt about it. But what happens after that is the problem. We can only go so far with willpower, and as soon as we get the body we've dreamed about, most of us run out of willpower and eat the foods that caused the weight gain in the first place more frequently. Since our belief about the consumption of the food we restricted didn't change, we eventually return to them.

When experts say that they have the perfect diet for you, they set you up for failure by making you believe you need to look for the best diet plan, and when you find it, you will live happily ever after. Off-the-shelf diets require you to change so much, usually recommending a very different nutrition plan than you are used to. You use your willpower to keep going, and it takes a lot of mental energy. When you blindly follow a process that an expert or a coach told you to, you are likely to fail eventually. Even though most likely they know more than you about diets and body transformation, you are the only person who can know what's best for you and your body. Fat loss and weight management is your process, not somebody else's protocol.

Insight 1: Willpower-Based Diets
Don't Work in the Long Run

I am sure you get excited when you start a new diet plan. I did this for so many years—actually, for decades. As time passes and it gets hard, you may think, "Screw it!" It is too hard, and you start eating whatever you want. You feel guilty and ashamed, and you beat yourself up for failing again. You think you just need to be even more disciplined, and you promise yourself you will be. Let's be honest: Most of us do this. We all use willpower, self-criticism, and restrictions to get results. What do a yo-yo diet and weight cycling having in common? They're essentially the same thing. When weight cycling is the result of on-and-off dieting, it's called yo-yo dieting.

Dieting can help you lose weight quickly; that's certain. Each of today's popular diets offers the same potential outcome as the next. Almost any diets that put you in a caloric deficit will give you short-term results. This type of weight loss is easy but not sustainable. Having enough willpower can result in sticking to diets, and this yields optimal results. I know for sure that sticking to a diet is a far greater determinant of successful weight loss than the type of diet the person stuck to. Even the best diet is a waste of time and energy because it takes willpower, which ends at some point, and then women and girls must search for the next quick plan. Neuroscientist Sandra Aamodt said in her TED Talk titled "Why Dieting Doesn't Usually Work" that this is because, "It relies on willpower, and as willpower is limited, any strategy that relies on its consistent application is pretty much guaranteed to eventually fail you when your attention moves on to something else. Willpower is exhaustible since it relies on self-control and forcing yourself. And this kind of change can never stick."

Insight 2: Diets Push You to Feel
Ashamed and Afraid of Food

Willpower-based diets have rules that you need to follow. These requirements are not about your psychological preferences. Therefore, diets don't help you make peace with food. They teach you to think about it as your enemy, and it works. Many of you beautiful ladies are afraid of food. It is mind-blowing if you think about it. In fact, you might be more afraid of food than anything else. You see it as something that gets in the way of your happiness and success. You can spend days after days in misery if you eat what you were not supposed to.

The diet mind-set creates shame around food, and we have a tendency to put our self-worth on the line for not eating the right thing. It makes me sad when I hear girls talking about their struggle after eating something that wasn't on the approved food list; they are just so hard on themselves. We think we are doing the right thing when we are on track with our food intake, but peace around food is nowhere to be found. We are so hung up on doing the next right thing that we lose the enjoyment of food.

The culture of dieting and weight loss is good at making value judgments about what we put in our mouth. And as soon as there is a value judgment attached to it, two major issues are created:

- Food gets divided into good and bad categories, and the diet-binge cycle arises.
- Our self-esteem and self-worth are based on how we eat and whether we eat only the foods that we are supposed to.

Unfortunately, when food is judged like this, you will associate food with guilt, shame, and embarrassment, even when you are not on a diet.

Insight 3: Dieting Doesn't Create a Long-Term Lifestyle

Diets target weight loss by eliminating food groups, particular macronutrients (protein, carbs or fat). The most recent popular plans are the Ketogenic and the Paleo (paleolithic) diets. They work and create fat loss. There are millions of people losing weight every day. As a professional nutritionist, it makes me happy and angry at the same time that there are countless advertisements about new ways to lose fat or weight. This is not our problem anymore. Our problem is with knowing how to keep it off. Most people who lose weight will put it back on within a couple of weeks or months. More often than not, they will gain so much that they weigh more than before they started the diet. There is an easy explanation for this: Because the way they lost the weight was not based on lifestyle changes but on restrictions, when they no longer aimed for weight loss, they didn't know how to keep the weight from reappearing. We have been conditioned to believe that diets are magical formulas for weight loss, and in a way, they are. They have a magic pill component to make you lose weight quickly, but they also have a Band-Aid component. That is, they often don't solve the issues that caused you to gain weight in the first place. And that means the weight will come back again. That's why diets are fads. They promise you something that a lot of us can get. But they also direct you to a dead end with weight management, because diets are not sustainable; they don't teach you sufficient new skills for what to do after you have lost weight.

Insight 4: Overindulgence in Food and Compulsive Eating Is Directly Related to Deprivation, Thanks to Dieting

After every diet, there is a binge. Diets don't regard social and cultural interactions. As mentioned previously, what diets do favor is separating food between good and bad and building shame and guilt around eating. Diets are very good at that, in fact. They also push us to overeat and binge on food. Cheat meals are the worst because they create a psychological mess. When you exclude large varieties of food from your diet, you might lose weight, but you also develop an unhealthy relationship with food. This is one way eating disorders thrive. When you are on diets, at some point you will cycle between restricting and binging on food, also called crash dieting. They offer the ultimate temptation, a quick fix. But when the body's compensatory mechanism kicks in, you can't maintain your diet anymore, and the deprivation you have created ultimately pushes you to binge on food.

Insight 5: The Diet Mentality Sends the Message That You Are Flawed

Whether you are conscious of it or not, the message you give yourself by jumping on the diet wagon is that until you get a new body, you have to put your life on hold. You believe you can't do what you want until you reach physical perfection; only then will everything be different. You will be more confident, and people will look at you differently. When you jump on the diet bandwagon, you acknowledge silently that this time, by pushing, controlling, shaming, restricting, and torturing yourself enough, somehow you will arrive happy and confident. However, when you get your new body, in many cases you realize you still have your insecurities or fears, and people don't change magically around you. Even though your body has changed, you might be afraid of gaining the weight back, so you judge, criticize fear, and punish yourself again to stay in shape. The fear behind dieting is unseen, but it is in every corner of the thoughts you have and decisions you make while you are on the diet bandwagon.

The Triggers of All Problems
Reason #2: Live by the Model of Eat Less, Exercise More

Most chronic dieters eat increasingly less to lose or manage their weight, and many of them are also chronic cardio exercisers. Are you one of them? If yes, this is not your fault. You were given this method as a solution time and time again. Unfortunately, it doesn't work. That's one reason you are reading this. Most of us habitually count calories and spend one to two hours on the cardio machine daily or at least a couple of times per week. I'm sure you have had success in the past, but you must be exhausted from this sort of plan. Your body might look thinner than it used to but not necessarily better.

The Connection Between Calories and Hormones

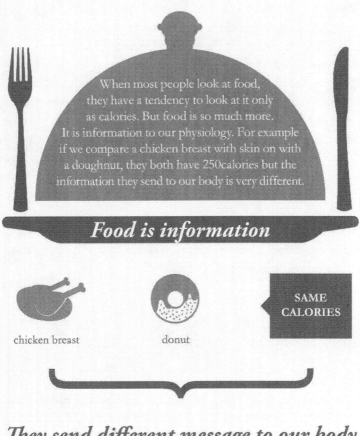

When most people look at food, they have a tendency to look at it only as calories. But food is so much more. It is information to our physiology. For example if we compare a chicken breast with skin on with a doughnut, they both have 250 calories but the information they send to our body is very different.

Food is information

chicken breast

donut

SAME CALORIES

They send different message to our body

Because of new discoveries in nutrition science in the last ten years, we have learned so much about how calories affect our hormones. Food eventually influences the fat burning or fat storage capacity of your body. As your five senses interact with and respond to your environment, your nervous system communicates with your endocrine system, a series of glands and tissues constantly at work manufacturing, delivering, and processing a wide assortment of hormones to maintain balance in your body. Hormones are chemical messengers between the body and the brain. Feeling the need to sleep, eat, or grab a coffee can be tracked back to the hormonal activity in your body. Hormones can also dictate where your body stores fat and how it releases it.

Therefore, based on the food you eat, you can put your body into a fat-burning or fat-storing mode. A doughnut or a piece of chicken could send very different messages to your body, both in terms of blood sugar regulation and storing or burning fat, as these foods contain very different amounts of fat, carbs, and protein.

Because of their connection with processing calories, hormones directly affect your appearance. They influence not only the look and feel of your skin or hair but also body composition. Hormones control your appetite and stimulate metabolism, so achieving and maintaining hormonal balance plays an essential role in achieving lasting weight loss.

Insight 1: Eating Less by Cutting Calories Causes Hormonal Chaos

When you suddenly cut calories to lose weight, several things can happen in your body:

- Since your body has a set point, within a range of ten or fifteen pounds, where it feels comfortable, out-of-control calorie cutting will make you feel hungrier because your body responds to restricted caloric intake by releasing hormones that stimulate appetite
- Your level of thyroid hormones drops, causing a slowdown in your metabolism
- Your level of stress hormone (cortisol) increases in response to the physical stress of skipping a meal or ingesting insufficient carbohydrate, which ultimately triggers insulin release
- It increases the hunger hormone ghrelin to stimulate appetite
- It decreases the satiety hormone called leptin, which decreases appetite, increases calorie burning, and regulates the amount of fat stored in the body

If your hormones are thrown into a state of chaos, your tendency to overeat kicks in. When your caloric intake starts to yo-yo in addition, your metabolism suffers a dangerous series of highs and lows. The end result includes weight gain (exactly what you did not want), cravings, mood imbalances, and a damaged metabolism. Most importantly, extreme caloric restrictions are not an effective long-term solution because they're not sustainable. The short-term victories achieved with this type of eating are always followed with rebound weight gain because, whether we like it or not, hormones kick in to return the body to its status quo. This is why following excessive caloric restrictions makes you want to eat more and more.

Calories and Insulin

Biochemically speaking, no matter whether carbs are processed and filled with chemicals or not, they all contain sugar. And the amount of sugar you eat has an effect on weight management. When you eat beans, legumes, sweet potatoes, fruits, or veggies, which are promoted as healthy, your digestive system breaks them down. After digestion, the body uses the vitamins and minerals to keep your body healthy and uses the derived sugar to give you energy.

The level of insulin in our bodies is mostly based on the carbohydrates we eat. Insulin's main job is to take nutrients out of your bloodstream and carry them to your cells to be used up. The more carbs you eat, the more insulin you will have in your body. This is because insulin also lowers blood sugar when it is above a healthy range.

A traditional breakfast might only be three hundred calories, but if you eat whole-grain cereal with milk, oatmeal with blueberries, or whole-grain toast and peanut butter with freshly squeezed orange juice, your body can't do anything but store some of it as fat. If you are taking in too many carbs and the body can't use it for energy, it will process the sugar into fat and store it in your fat cells. This is worth repeating: Carbohydrates turn into sugar in the body after digestion, and if the amount of sugar from the carbs you eat doesn't get used up with the help of insulin, your body will store the rest as fat, even if your meals are low in calories.

Therefore, successful weight management is not about eating less but eating smarter. Understand the impact food has on your body, and use it to your advantage.

Insight 2: Long Steady-State Cardio Is Not an Effective Weight-Loss Tool

Just like food has an impact on our fat-burning or fat-storing hormones, so does exercise. Most of us don't know that cardio has a different effect on burning fat than weight training does. In the last two decades, fitness professionals and body builders recommended lots of steady-state cardio to lose or manage weight. We took this advice seriously, and many of us spent not just one but two hours on the cardio machine per day. We had thin appearances but no muscle definition. We might look great in clothes, but how did we look underneath? Now, think about people who sprint or do strength training. Their bodies are much more toned. You can only do an hour or two of cardio per day, and you can't keep it up the rest of your life. Once your body is used to this type of calorie burning, you will most likely gain weight before long if you change your routine. Learn to work out smarter, not harder. For fat loss, intensity trumps duration.

Most people who struggle with weight and are willing to exercise think, "I'll just do cardio until I lose weight, and then I might add weights to tone up later." When I worked as a personal trainer for a couple of years, I heard most women say that they didn't do weight training because they were afraid of bulking up. This couldn't be further from the truth. Adding weight training to your exercise regimen helps you lose fat faster, and you lose fat instead of muscle. In contrast, doing cardio alone burns calories, but when you stop, the caloric burn stops, and you could be losing muscle as well, making you fatter at the end.

Fat loss and weight loss are two very different concepts. You can lose weight pretty easily if greatly reduce how much you eat and do a lot of cardio every day. You will lose a ton of muscles in the process, and when you stop this lifestyle and resume your old eating and activity patterns, you will experience the yo-yo effect of weight gain immediately.

Cardio queens, pay attention here: The more cardio you do, the less your body responds over time, and you have to keep doing more simply to maintain. You have probably noticed this happen before. This can only show the relationship between food and body transformation. This is why cleaning up your food intake is more important than the number of hours you spend on the treadmill.

The Triggers of All Problems
Reason #3: Emotional Appetite

Most professionals—including weight-loss coaches, personal trainers, dietitians, and doctors—accuse diets as the root cause of chronic weight struggles. The major part of their work is to create a diet plan to give quick results or a long-term nutrition plan from which, slowly but surely, people have a lifelong plan for achievable weight loss. Even personal trainers recognize more and more that you can't out train a bad diet and that you must be educated in nutrition as well.

I believe there is a second major component to chronic dieting and ongoing weight struggles that often gets ignored or isn't recognized among professionals, which is *compulsive eating.*

We all love to eat. Food is not only for survival but also for fuel. Enjoying food is one of the most beautiful experiences we can have on earth. It is a cultural experience that we share. A meal can add pleasure to our lives. And it is a delightful experience that can be combined with social gatherings.

Children and adults all eat emotionally and use food as a tranquilizer from time to time, and that's fine. Occasionally we all eat when we are not physically hungry because food enhances our life on a personal and social level. What a great feeling to have an afternoon with a great friend or spend some time with a family member in your favorite store to get a pastry or yummy sweets.

But for many people, their relationship to food has changed, and food has power over them. They use and overuse food as a way of coping, and sooner or later, people use it to deal with their emotions. It is a source of pleasure and joy, but at the same time, food brings up guilt and shame. This becomes a problem when you use food as a constant life enhancer. You are affected not only when you are hit by feelings of guilt and shame around eating but also in how you see your body as a basis to your happiness as your weight becomes an issue. Food is very soothing because it changes our body chemistry and hormones and eventually how we feel. When you eat for nourishment and for the love of food, which gives you pleasure and joy, your relationship to eating is what it is supposed to be. Even if you eat to ward off a bad mood or give yourself something as a reward, it is fine.

There is a huge difference between occasionally fixing your mood with food, doing it compulsively, and choosing food as a dominant coping mechanism to deal with different emotional states.

Certain things may trigger emotions that make you feel you need to zone out on food. It becomes a problem when food is overused to cope with or avoid feelings.

Emotional eating patterns are actually a mechanism of the mind and emotions. When you are at peace with yourself, you are at peace with food, but when emotions arise that you can't handle, your appetite rises too.

Brad Yates says, "Self-sabotage is simply misguided self-love."

The problem is not about you lacking willpower and discipline to eat the right thing or the right amount. It is about your emotions making you eat compulsively, a representation of your limited ability to take care of yourself otherwise.

This is what I call "reactive eating." It is not necessarily caused by life-changing experiences or traumas. When I was working as a fitness manager in Manhattan, I had the chance to interview more than six hundred people about their weight struggles. I picked up on the ones who where chronic dieters with ongoing weight struggles, and we dug deeper. When I asked how their eating could be impacted by their moods, most would talk about emotional eating in the midst of feeling tired, feeling down, or being sleep deprived, so they looked to food for a pick-me-up. This made me realize that emotional eating doesn't always mean a deep psychological matter requiring therapy. It often originates from basic human needs and is caused by stress, anxiety, or fear because of things such as the following:

- Unmet needs for fun, play, excitement, or recreation
- A desire for love, affection, appreciation, and romance
- Anger, resentment, disappointment, bitterness, frustration, or emptiness
- Fear of uncertainty, fear of insecurity, or a desire for comfort
- Low energy, too much work, and not enough play

When different emotions arise based on circumstances, reactive eaters can respond to these emotions by grabbing whatever food feels like it will take away the feeling that they can't always identify but certainly don't want to feel. The food will always be very sweet, fatty, or salty in these circumstances. Based on my professional experience throughout the years, reactive eating can be triggered by anything. The sky is the limit. However, the following is a list of the most prevalent thoughts and emotions I came across that triggered reactive eating:

- Constantly thinking about body image insecurities like never being thin, lean, strong, or skinny enough
- Being hyper aware of lack of anything
- Having unmet needs
- Having emotional pain
- Thinking negative, critical, fearful, and self-defeating thoughts
- Struggling with shame and the fear being insufficient
- Feeling you don't know where you end and others begin; carrying the weight of the world

- Feeling imperfect
- Being anxious
- Suppressing anger, resentment
- Having unresolved pain from childhood or past experiences related to family, friends, and teachers
- Dealing with self-esteem issues
- Experiencing daily stress
- Feeling stuffed down and not expressed
- Feeling you can't express the truth of who you are
- Seeking fulfillment
- Desiring love, affection, appreciation, or romance
- Using food as a substitute for affection
- Not admitting to yourself or others what you truly desire
- Yearning for closeness, love, being held and simulating the comfort via food
- Feeling insecurity
- Feeling powerless
- Having unexpressed emotions
- Feeling different or not fitting in
- Experiencing happiness anxiety
- Feeling disconnected
- Having a general sense of purposelessness
- Feeling weight stigma, vulnerability about body shape

Some food cravings are about emotions that surface in the moment, but many others are deeply rooted in beliefs and emotions.

So, emotional eating is mostly compulsive and chronic behavior based upon reactions, triggered by overwhelming feelings. Your eating is not based on true physical hunger. Instead, you engage in emotional eating when there is a split second that you feel so unsafe that you believe the ground is gone, and you look for ways to get back on your feet again and balance yourself mentally and emotionally. You choose food to help. Your eating serves you at the moment, but at the end, you feel guilty or ashamed. Do you ever wonder why you always lose some—if not all—of the weight you gain back or why you gain weight back when you lost it before?

Some of your answers are probably similar to the following:

- When I gained weight, I felt lonely, bored, busy, stressed out, and unmotivated to have better eating habits.
- I had too much fun partying and spending time with friends, including social eating. I got a new boyfriend, and I was so happy that I couldn't stop eating.
- I lost weight because I wanted to look better so I was liked more by others and myself. I wanted to look more beautiful. I realized being thinner meant I could get more attention and more happiness in my life.

Chronic weight fluctuation, weight cycling, and unsuccessful weight management don't necessarily happen because we don't know what we need to do to care for ourselves and manage our weight. Almost all people whose weight fluctuates understand the importance of exercise, sleep, and stress reduction. However, you can know everything there is to know about eating healthily and yet your weight fluctuates. You experience moments, days, and weeks when your emotions don't lead you to eating in a healthy manner or taking good care of yourself. When emotions are just too much to handle, you need something to cuddle up with to calm you down. You use food for your soul, as you don't feel alignment with yourself; zoning out from your life by eating compulsively feels like a must. And then when you somehow find peace in your life, your appetite naturally dissipates.

Compulsive eating happens when you are not tuned in with your body and mind, and you think you are hungry but you actually are not. If you are not aware of the mood and food connection, you might truly believe that when you want to eat something sweet or fatty, you are really hungry. Your mind goes haywire, and you lose your sanity around food despite your best efforts. You might have just finished a full meal, but you want to eat more. You can't help overeating or binging on food. These are clues that you eat in response to emotions instead of real hunger. And the more you do it, the more it becomes a habit of dealing with emotions this way.

Compulsive eating is an umbrella term for emotional eating based on reactive eating induced by thoughts, beliefs, or emotions. In order to move through your feelings, you lean on binge eating, numbing, overeating, emotional eating, or mood eating as a means to distract yourself. It can take the form of eating alone or among people, but the bottom line is taking the edge off of a feeling you can't handle.

Many of us think that we simply have to be more in control, have a better regimen, have more discipline, and so on. Chronic dieters stuck in a loop of doing the same thing over and over again don't realize that in order to stop the self-destructive pattern, they need to pay attention to more than what they put in their mouth. They also need to understand why they are choosing food at certain moments.

If you don't pay attention, you run the risk of turning your habits into an autopilot. In certain situations, like when you are stressed out, anxious, happy, sad, tired, or when you feeling unfulfilled, you will eat without even thinking about it. This happens because numbing out on food is always about experiencing relief to help you get back on your feet.

How and Why We Numb Out on Food

Most people's immediate reaction when asked to admit they might have addictions or compulsive issues around food can be tricky because emotional eating is not clinically considered a legitimate addiction. We make a strong distinction between people who legitimately suffer from addictions to drugs, alcohol, and gambling and healthy people. But there are a lot of us in the less defined middle who struggle with compulsive behaviors to a chronic extent, and they get in the way of our living life to its full potential. Compulsive behaviors are great for allowing us to hide from our vulnerabilities. Whether they involve watching TV for hours and feeling drained afterward or numbing out on food, these behaviors are great ways to hide behind something so that we don't have to engage in our life. It is easy to do, and numbing isn't officially recognized as a compulsive behavior interfering with our emotional, mental, or physical health.

Elaborating upon earlier sections of this chapter, you engage in emotional eating because a deep internal need for emotional protection exists. You try to run away from your feelings, as you live in a world of insecurity; hence, you carry emotional weight.

The method of engaging in emotional eating is different at different times. It might take the form of binging, craving, mindless indulging, emotional eating, overeating, or numbing (zoning) out on food. As mentioned previously, any kind of compulsive eating can take place alone or in social surroundings.

Most of the time, "binge eating" is a phrase used in the context of eating alone and hiding from people. The term "overeating" is usually used to refer to behavior in social gatherings, but you can absolutely engage in overeating when alone. Another aspect of the term "compulsive eating" means not only that you eat when you are not physically hungry but that the amount of food and the frequency of eating is a lot. The speed of your eating is also relevant. In compulsive eating, you eat really fast, and you barely chew or enjoy the taste of your food.

Although there is no strict definition for who belongs to this group, there are some distinct sources of emotional hunger all driven by different types of trigger points, which may be conscious or subconscious. Lasting change occurs when you can clarify what you really crave and fill that unmet need. Some reasons might be applicable to you, and some won't be. Battling even one can be difficult. I am going to identify sixteen types of reactive eating. When you eat at these times, you are not physically hungry and are therefore eating beyond your physical needs.

Why We Numb Out on Food

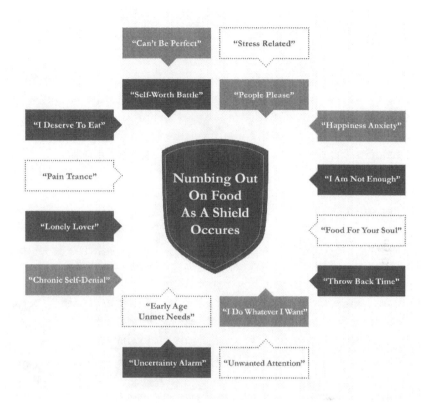

I Deserve to Eat

You have too much to do in your life, and you feel you deserve to wind down with food and get inspired with bouts of emotional eating.

Can't Be Perfect

Many times, women put one aspect of their lives ahead of every other. It's like saying that to be successful in one thing, other aspects need to suffer. This can lead to feeling a lack in one aspect of your life so great that you try to overcompensate it with food. Weight management is an important goal for you, but without respecting the body, you are sabotaging yourself with emotional eating.

Stress-Related Eating

At times of emotional stress, food can be used as a tool to manage stress. Stress sometimes brings out overwhelming feelings, but when the perceived danger is gone, you overeat. Basically, the emotional state overrides the appetite, and then after depriving yourself of food, there is a straight line to overeat when the hunger signals come back.

Happiness Anxiety

A lot of times, compulsive eating has a reputation to be used only when we experience negative emotions, but this is not the reality. A lot of people can binge when experiencing happy feelings as well. Subconsciously, food is used as a means to enhance the happiness before it disappears. In this type of emotional eating, food is not about pleasure and cultural experience but preventing the void that might be coming up later, as happiness is unconsciously seen as a limited resource. This type of compulsive eating can happen when you are alone, or you might be a social emotional eater who enjoys social gathering so much that you overindulge in food while you are bonding with friends. There is a point when you use food to enhance happy feelings without respecting your body's needs.

Pain Trance

You have strong emotions that don't go away within a short period of time—boredom, depression, grief, depression, anxiety, or sadness—and you have difficulty moving past or working through them. You store your feelings inside of you, and you choose the refrigerator to numb them out. Food distracts you from these feelings. This is a mindless way of disconnecting not only from yourself but from the act of eating. You don't pay attention to food during the process. Once you are done, you realize you didn't savor the bites. You judge yourself and feel ashamed as you come back to awareness.

Self-Worth Battle

If you take things very personally, and your self-esteem or self-worth highly depends on what other people think of you or how they treat you, you may numb your feelings to avoid confrontation. When you feel somebody is taking advantage of you or belittling you, instead of creating boundaries and standing up for yourself, you numb with food. Because of a lack of self-nurturing skills, you tend to be hard on yourself, and eating is just another way to mistreat yourself.

People Pleaser

When there is tension in your close relationships, you feel like numbing with food to avoid feelings of disappointment, anger, or fear of rejection. You prefer to give people what they want from you, so instead of standing up for yourself, you binge on food to get some emotional relief. You don't think you can express the truth of your identity, and then your feelings are being stuffed down instead of expressed. A longstanding relationship of emotional trauma can affect this type of emotional eating.

I Am Not Enough

This type of eating happens when you are hypercritical of yourself, and you compare your mistakes and failures to your image of what you are supposed to be. Your subconscious belief tells you that you are not enough, and the gap between the expectations and where you see yourself creates rebellion. Emotional eating is a way of giving yourself some love. You quickly label yourself stupid, loser, or bad as a means to attack yourself. You eat to stuff down your lack of self-acceptance and self-love.

Lonely Lover

Your hunger is activated because you miss intimacy or are feeling lonely in your love relationship. Your basic needs for security and trust are perhaps not being met. You are seeking love and fulfillment, but you are somehow convinced that it will not come to you, so you use food as a substitute for affection. You crave closeness and the feeling of being loved, hugged, and held. Again, you don't get it, so you subconsciously stimulate the feeling of closeness by eating and feel good for a short period of time.

Early Unmet Needs

Perhaps you didn't learn self-nurturing skills as a child, so you end up using food as a Band-Aid to address childhood wounds. You want to take care of yourself, but without the right skills, food is your route to feeling carefree.

I Do Whatever I Want

When you feel overwhelmed by the pressure and rules life puts on you, you want to feel independent from the applied structures and not worry about anything. So, you eat, do, or say anything you are not supposed to reject expectations.

Food for Your Soul

Overeating, binging, and numbing your feelings with food can represent your depleted soul and the attempt to fill an inner void. You may feel empty, bored, unmotivated, uninspired, or uneasy; you might have a sense of longing for more in life, feel a lack of personal fulfillment or desires, feel disconnected, or have a general sense of being lost in life. Perhaps you lack purpose or meaningful activities and miss nourishing connections. You choose food to replace your emptiness so that you don't have to feel.

Chronic Self-Denial

When you deny yourself of what you truly want and who you truly are, you are ultimately depriving yourself from your desires. You do this because somewhere deep inside of you, you don't believe you deserve what you want, so you punish yourself. Since your belief is so deeply rooted and is related to limiting beliefs, although you experience an internal starvation in many areas, you take it out on food by disowning your body's signals of hunger and fullness.

Uncertainty Alarm

As life throws challenging situations at you, your appetite kicks in to soothe your fear of failure, fear of uncertainty, and feelings of insecurity. To avoid worrying, food helps you calm down like a security blanket.

Unwanted Attention

Many times, women and girls consciously want to get thin and sexy. But when they get noticed for their body, they feel uncomfortable and subconsciously override their desire to stay in shape, so they start eating more to get away from this attention. We feel safer when we use our weight as an excuse to hide instead of shining. When we lose weight, compliments can trigger unwanted attention. We can feel violated by the way a man looks at us or feel ashamed by enjoying the attention of others.

Payback Time

Emotional or psychological wounds like rejection, resentment, unforgiveness, failure, guilt, or shame can trigger a syndrome wherein you stuff yourself with food to pay back those who have hurt you. It is like using your own body as a battleground to work out issues or settle the emotional pain you suffer. You essentially use food to transform feelings and emotions. In fact, you don't know what to do with the actual feeling, so you use food for comfort.

I wonder how many of you are aware when you are eating to seek comfort and not based on true physical hunger. Can you identify when you are triggered to engage in emotional eating behavior? Do you recognize any of your eating patterns just described? How would you feel if you had to give up the habit of eating when your emotions trigger it?

The following signs can also help you understand whether you eat emotionally:

- You keep eating, grazing, or nibbling because you can't figure out what you are truly hungry for.
- When you are physically hungry, any food is good enough, but with emotional eating, there's a specific food in mind you need to have.
- You feel the desire to eat above your neck—in your mind and your mouth—and sometimes in your heart, but definitely not in your stomach. Hunger, to you, represents a strong emotion, not biological hunger.
- After you are done eating, you don't remember tasting the food.
- You eat to the point of physical discomfort. You want to stop, but you can't.
- Hunger comes in a split second. One moment, you aren't thinking about food, and then all you can think about is food and consuming it.

How We Numb Out on Food

Jennie Kramer, a New York City psychotherapist and the director and founder of Metro Behavioral Health Associates says that emotional appetite is usually categorized by three different types of behaviors:

- **Emotional Eating:** This can be triggered by some sort of episode or occurrence, and it can be done in public or in secret.
- **Compulsive Overeating:** People graze all day and then eat whatever is put in front of them later in the day. It's also done in public or in secret.
- **Binge Eating:** It is often done in secrecy. We don't want other people to see that we are eating.

Food is not the main issue. I wasn't really conscious of my relationship to food in terms of numbing or overeating. I truly felt that when I wanted to eat, I was physically hungry. After learning more about it, I didn't know how I would treat myself after a long day at work if food wasn't an option.

Is Dieting or Emotional Eating a Coping Mechanism?

Food isn't something that should scare you. If you are scared, you have work to do. Emotional eating and dieting are products of your thoughts, beliefs, and emotions.

Being a chronic dieter is based on an unspoken fear of not getting the job you want, not getting a husband, not having friends, or not getting a life you truly want and desire. You believe that if you could just stay on a diet, you would eventually end up with a new body and a new life. And then everything would be peaceful and ideal, giving you ultimate happiness.

Eating when you are not physically hungry in the form of compulsive eating, including overeating, binge eating, or numbing out on food, is a product of you feeling disconnected from life. As discussed previously, you are trying to meet a need that is not related to food. If you are aware of your compulsive eating pattern, it can help you discover something else is going on in your life.

The only way to effectively deal with an ongoing pattern of dieting or emotional eating is to not look at it as a terrible thing. Focusing on how bad it is and how you should avoid it is not very productive. I invite you to instead focus on the underlying reasons for why you want to diet all the time or eat compulsively. As you focus on what's going on behind the habit and come up with solutions, you will naturally move away from wanting to be on diets continuously or eating emotionally because you have dismantled the reason.

Emotionally eating or being a chronic dieter is not inherently bad; it is a coping mechanism. Unfortunately, it can get in the way of living your life fully and being able to manage your weight. But if you look at the bigger picture, it is not the worst thing happening to you. I hope you get some relief by realizing that even though ongoing dieting or emotional eating are symptoms of the evil and struggles in your life, understanding what else is going on is the first step to real and lasting changes.

Even though recognized addictions such as alcohol, drugs, or gambling are considered to be the things that need to be removed, they are also often engaged in for underlying reasons. Some people would say that you are addicted to drugs, gambling, or alcohol the same way you are addicted to food. I believe that any chronic and compulsive behaviors we engage in have an underlying cause for why we are doing it, not because we are addicted to the thing itself. There is a point when you can look at numbing behaviors related to drugs, food, or gambling as an addiction to the substance, but if you take a step back and look at the issue from a holistic point of view, you realize we do things that feel good not only to enjoy life but also to avoid pain or emotions we can't handle, and so we avoid life.

Diets are based on the belief that if you engage in them, you have the opportunity to prove yourself worthy of anything.

As a nutritionist, I used to let my clients to have cheat days to prevent going crazy around food. I now firmly believe this is a big mistake. It took me some time to realize it, but restricting will always lead to cheating in general. This is because when you have a mind-set of not being able to have something, you also have the implication that when you have the thing, its purpose is to calm and comfort you, and this creates a bad relationship with food overall.

You've Experienced Constant Fear, Loneliness, and Insecurity

We like to use coping mechanisms in the following sorts of situations:

- When the pain is too big for us to handle
- When we are not able to change our situation
- When the pain we are in is more comfortable than changing the situation

Interestingly enough, in our society, we learn to deal with physical injury by taking it easy for a while. You know you need to rest, and the people around you may even feel compassion toward you. However, emotional or psychological injuries never really get talked about in the same way.

Emotional injuries are things like abandonment, attacks, loneliness, neglect, rejection, weight stigmas and body shame, unexpressed emotions, unfulfillment, fear of uncertainty, low self-worth or self-esteem, losing someone we love, and so on. Like physical traumas, emotional injuries create wounds and leave us with invisible scars. And psychological traumas essentially force us to cope with emotional injuries in the form of anxiety, fear, depression, sadness, shame, or guilt. These are the invisible force behind our emotional eating patterns.

For people whose weight fluctuates all the time, it won't work to only fix their diets. If we only focus on nutrition and replace one diet with another nutrition plan, it's not going to help remove the disordered eating behavior, emotional eating. Many girls and women who struggle with reactive eating believe that when they get thinner, their unhappiness will be removed magically. However, if we don't address feelings of unworthiness or lack of self-love, and if we don't become aware of the underlying beliefs that trigger these feelings, permanent weight loss and peace of mind will not be within reach. They will remain a desire.

If you struggle with compulsive dieting or compulsive eating in any form, you need to unblock the root cause. And the only way to do this is feeling what you feel instead of eating what you feel.

The habits of dieting or reactive eating are so incredibly ingrained that it feels like the habit (binge eating or numbing) simultaneously controls you and gives you a feeling of power. Looking for relief from life's craziness is not unusual, but we need to look somewhere other than food. The goal is to make a conscious decision to get to the bottom of the issue.

Compulsive eaters hate their binges and overeating patterns. Not in the moment, necessarily, but definitely afterward. We want to get rid of this habit so that we can move on with our lives. We often say, "I am sick of this," or, "I wonder if this issue with food will ever go away." Well, the moving on part is definitely possible, but you can't skip any steps. Dealing with weight fluctuation is very hard way to live indeed. It's like a constant struggle to do the right things, and when we don't, we feel disconnected from life. Diet books, weight-loss gurus, and personal trainers miss the point when they try to solve emotional eating, overeating, and binges by focusing on food. It's not about what you eat but why you eat.

There are endless stories for why we eat emotionally, but it is not because we don't have enough discipline or self-control. It is about working with the issue from the inside. Emotional eating is not causing the problem. Stop thinking about it this way. Emotional eating is the effect. Seek to understand it instead. If you want to address the problem, you need to solve the root cause. You can't fill your emotions with something—food—that was not designed for that purpose. Things you eat can give you temporary good feelings, but they will never resolve emotional issues in the long run.

How many times have you experienced feeling fine in one moment, and then you suddenly wanted to have ice cream, a bag of chips, or chocolate as quickly as possible? Part of emotional eating is absolutely subconscious; it is a behavior you've conditioned yourself to do.

Having the desire to consume no food can be compulsive as well, and it can lead to anorexia. You might not be aware of what you are feeling or why you are eating or not eating, but simply put, something inside of you needs to be filled.

Sometimes the emotional pain can be so strong or so buried that even when emotional nourishment is offered, you are not able to accept it. Choosing food seems safer trusting someone or opening up.

Food is less dangerous than drugs or alcohol as a means to transfer emotions, but it can lead you to weight struggles. These, in turn, seem to control your mind, your confidence, and the way you show up in your life. Underneath the overeating or undereating, there is a longing to love and to be loved. The illusion of having control over food gives you counterfeit love. It is not real, but in the moment, it satisfies your needs.

There is nothing wrong about wanting to feel good. Everybody has this goal, but using food as a substance to feel good is more about escaping from an issue. Most of us have some form of attachment to things to sense relief, whether playing video games, watching TV, playing a sport, or surfing the net to zone out and put aside our feelings. Other people are workaholics, using work to numb out their emotions. I am not suggesting that you choose other types of numbing behaviors instead of food. I am just pointing out that we all have some form of them. You are not alone. The object of the compulsive behavior is almost irrelevant; what's more important is what lies behind the compulsion. What are you covering up or denying with this behavior?

Experiencing emotions like love, fear, joy, or sadness can make you realize whether you have the skill and self-connection to handle or express your emotions without reaching for food or any other numbing behavior. Thoughts and feelings flow within us all the time; this comes with being a human. But if you're an emotional eater, you react to your thoughts and emotions by using food to get realigned with yourself—to get centered. You are desperate to take the edge off of a feeling and to feel content. Without using food to convey feelings, you can't function. Reactive eaters need to find a way to stop using food when they are in emotional turmoil. Although reactive eating is what makes you binge and gain weight, it is actually a protective coping mechanism.

We've discussed how food obsessions like dieting, thinking about food all the time, cravings for food when you are not hungry, binge eating, overeating, or other compulsory eating patterns that ultimately result in weight issues are just a consequence of whatever else you are truly hungry for.

If you keep covering up your emotions with food, it's like putting an adhesive bandage on a deep wound. It is important to understand that unless you are willing to work and understand what feelings lead you to overeating or binging to numb the emotional roller coaster inside of you, you cannot and will not reach permanent weight loss. Eating in response to happiness, sadness, anxiety, or boredom can't fill up your emotional needs. Instead, you need to address the root cause of you emotions that make you want to eat, as mentioned previously in this chapter. If you can look at your issue from this side, it means you are able to open up yourself to real transformation.

If we can step away from the idea that we are addicted to food and instead see that something else totally not connected to food wants attention, we might understand that our eating behaviors are here to protect, hide, or balance emotions we don't know how to feel. You could actually see it as a gift, as I started to during my transformation. If I hadn't gained weight, I might have never been aware and uncovered things that eventually helped me lead a much happier life.

Therefore, your compulsive eating patterns highlight your difficulty to connect with yourself and respond appropriately when you are out of balance emotionally, physically, mentally, or spiritually.

It is crucial to understand that it is not the feeling themselves that cause the binging, numbing, overeating, or compulsive eating. It is our attempts to keep from experiencing the feelings understanding them. We don't want to face why we have certain feelings. The main goal should not be to find something instead of eating so that we can have the body we want. Rather, we need to find the root cause of the reasons we feel the way we do and transform those issues so that we feel more aligned with who we are rather than jumping from one numbing behavior to another.

I hope it is clear by now that being unable to stay with your feelings without numbing out on food is as big of a deal as the fact that you do numb out on food and gain weight. I understand you are reading this to find a solution to your weight struggles and you want to have peace with food, but whether you can process your emotions is a much bigger deal. What are you ultimately after? Is it a perfect body or a deep inner peace no matter what emotions come up, allowing you to feel joy and happiness in the moment?

Emotional eating saves your sanity when it is happening. It is like sitting in a pitch-black room and feeling terrified by the dark, but when you light a candle, it feels soothing, exactly like food when you eat compulsively. When you blow the candle out, although you are left alone in the dark again, the lingering smell of the candle reminds you of the light. As it goes away, you find yourself in the pitch-black room again, terrified.

We've explored how emotional eating is a coping mechanism or skill. It is a behavioral habit that has worked for you up until now. But now that know better, you want to do better, right?

To get over emotional eating, first acknowledge the fact that eating for emotional nourishment is only a distraction from what's really going on inside of you. Emotional eating is a reaction to certain feelings. If you want to manage your weight and stop chronic weight fluctuations, your job is to work through emotions without pushing them down or numbing out on food. There is no way around this.

The good side of the story is that when you learn how to move through your feelings, you not only stop weight fluctuation but also go forward in your life. It might sound scary first since it takes courage to show up in your life. It all goes back to how badly you want to move forward and let go of chronic weight struggles.

When you are aware that your eating is based on reacting to emotions and has nothing to do with real physical hunger, you know you want to binge for the feelings to go away. Acknowledge the fact that you want to numb those feelings with food and perhaps hide from yourself.

The Triggers of All Problems
Reason #4: Trapped in Body Image Insecurity and Shame

Compulsive dieting is rooted in our lack of body acceptance. We feel terror, agitation, and stress about fat. Most of us who think we are fat consciously think there is something wrong with us. Lack of self-love and self-acceptance play a huge role in this mentality.

As diets push you to overeat and gain weight in the long run, more often than not, compulsive emotional eating also causes weight gain, and women and girls eventually have body image insecurities as well. This topic rarely gets talked about among professionals in the weight-loss industry, even though it holds the key for anyone with years of chronic struggles with dieting and weight management to move forward.

When women and girls restrict their food intake or go on diets, 99 percent of the time, the reason actually has more to do with trying to control something in their life, not their bodies. This can be a situation or a particular outcome we want to control. And because we fear losing control of the situation, we instead choose to control our body, either consciously or subconsciously.

Interestingly enough, we focus on controlling our weight to get control of our life. We try to control our weight to influence the outcome of applying for a job, being accepted by others, getting the guy we want, and so on.

So, food gets a lot of attention, but the real issue is what we want to control in our life, and food is the means to get it. When I worked as a fitness manager in Manhattan, I had the opportunity to ask hundreds of new members about certain issues. And when I asked what made them want to control or restrict their food intake, I came to the conclusion that we ultimately want to control what people think of us or how they respond to us. The bottom line was that I realized *we want to control our lovability*.

It sounds silly and simple, but it is the truth: We control how we look so that people will love us more. We believe that if we control how we look, people will be nicer to us.

Unfortunately until you see your value apart from having the perfect body, you will suffer. As long as you look for outside validation of your worth and lovability, you will struggle. Until you believe you only deserve to have the guy you want when you have the best body, you will always choose dieting instead of common sense and what you truly deserve.

The reality is this: When you put so much effort into staying in perfect shape, a guy might like the way you look better. But in reality, just because you are skinny, it doesn't mean everything will work out the way you want it to with him. It might get you in the door with someone, but controlling food to control your life is not the solution to your inner struggle to love yourself. Fear of the unknown is hard to deal with, but dieting and restricting food intake is not the ultimate solution to having self-acceptance and inner peace.

Influence of Familial, Cultural, and Media Messages

Our body image is a mental picture of how we think and feel about our physical body. Unfortunately, this image may have little to do with our actual appearance. There are social and cultural expectations for every single part of us—how we are supposed to look from our heads to our toes. Our body perception becomes loaded with these characteristics.

Body shame is so powerful and often so deeply rooted in our psyches that it affects women's ability to speak out with confidence about how we feel in many areas. These aspects of life can include career, health, motherhood, sexuality, life purpose, parenting, aging, and so on.

Body-image insecurity is a huge shame trigger for women because of the insecurity surrounding expectations to look smoking hot. Although we may be against those expectations, on some level we accept them as they are. And it hurts even more not to meet them, so we feel inadequate for being the way we are.

When our bodies fill us with disgust and feelings of unworthiness, shame can fundamentally change who we are and how we approach the world. When we blame and hate our bodies for failing to live up to expectations, we split ourselves and move away from our wholeness— our authentic, true self.

It's hard to find girls and women who are comfortable with their bodies. Do you value yourself and measure your worth based on what others think of your body's shape or appearance?

We put so much time and energy into making sure that we meet everyone's expectations that we are often left feeling angry, resentful, and fearful. Sometimes we turn these emotions inward and convince ourselves that we are bad indeed and that maybe we deserve the rejection that we so desperately fear. Shame is not reserved for the unfortunate few who have survived terrible traumas. It lurks in all of the familiar places, including appearance and body image.

When I was working in the TV industry in my twenties, the idea of false reality started to emerge. I was responsible for getting sponsors on different shows through product placement. I had ongoing relationships with about 150 different companies. I arranged for their products and services to appear in shows, and viewers could also win products.

I had an ongoing responsibility to make sure those prizes appeared in the show and targeted the audience. I always had to know how the prizes resonated with the viewers and so on. This taught me that people are sold a false reality through media.

I couldn't believe the impact I made on those people's lives by telling them what to fear—through product placement—so that they would realize a need to get particular products or services to make their life happier. I was just placing them in the show based on what people wanted to win, but the way the products were sold could give the impression to viewers that their life would be nothing without them.

I was shocked at how many people actually believe the media. But the experience also made me realize I was one of them, consuming all the messages targeting me—from lotion creams to give me nicer skin or a new diet pill to make me skinnier. Of course, I only reacted to those advertisements and sales pitches where I felt my skin was kind of dry or I felt I could lose a couple of pounds here and there. But would I have felt the need for those things if someone hadn't pointed them out as flaws? The conclusion I had about marketing and advertisements back then was that different types of beliefs can be deposited into people's minds after their psyche has been purposely disturbed with fear, joy, anger, excitement, or worry. As a result, there is higher possibility people will buy the advertised product or service to fix their emotional needs. Media is great for controlling the flow of information and creating emotional triggers so that people feel flawed and imperfect and then buy more products and services.

The Way We Think about Ourselves Starts When We Are Young

The experiences that affect how we perceive our bodies start in schools, when classmates tease girls who are flat-chested, fat, skinny, short, tall, or who have big boobs or big butts. Girls discover their power over boys and over their bodies as they realize that physical appearance can be a great tool for popularity. And being liked and popular seems more important than anything else.

Our perception is that once we lose weight, we will finally be happy and fulfilled as a person. We would look thin based on the current standards for look and shape considered desirable by others.

Instead of focusing on what we like about ourselves and what we desire, we instead focus on our desirability. While we are growing up, the media and social and cultural expectations influence us. We take our cues from them.

We find ourselves knowing more about how we are supposed to look, but those images and expectations have nothing to do with what happiness feels like for us.

To varying degrees, we all know the struggle to feel comfortable with ourselves in a society that puts so much importance on being perfect and fitting in. So, we try to fit in a box as being thin, beautiful, smart, and sexy is demanded of us.

Andrew Walen, psychotherapist and the executive director of the Body Image Therapy Center says in an interview that researchers have found that more often when a family member, teacher, a friend, or a significant other comments on someone's weight for weight-loss purposes, the greater the likelihood that person will turn to binge eating because of the shame and guilt she or he feels for his or her size. Our body-image issues started somewhere in the past. It may not be a weight stigma at first, but eventually it gets there.

The Real Reason Behind Wanting to Get Thin

When I asked people if they felt worthy with their "imperfect" bodies, they would choke up and say something like, "I am worthy of love, kind of, but I will be really worthy of it if I lose the last ten, twenty, or thirty pounds," or, "if I am able to maintain my weight, I will be really worthy of love."

Realizing the value our society places on beauty and thinness, it's not a big surprise that attractiveness is one of the most important assets into which people invest their sense of self-worth. We've been constantly told that being thin, having certain measurements, or reaching a particular number on the scale is direct proof of what we can expect regarding our success. It tells us to expect how many people will like us and whether we will be accepted or rejected. Images from the media remind us that if we were thin, we would be happy and accepted. Since most of us can't look exactly like the portrayed images, we are in an epic struggle to accept our bodies and ourselves.

Here is the truth: You don't want to be thin just to be told you are beautiful or that you have a great figure. You want all of these things to feel you are worth anything. And you want to be worthy so you can fit in anywhere in society. If people love you for these reasons, eventually you can accept and love yourself. You can feel like you are enough, and finally you will be happy.

The yo-yo effect of losing and gaining weight, chronic dieting, and emotions all play a huge part in our struggles for the perfect body, but in the meantime, our perceived worthiness is at stake.

The real driving force behind our weight-loss efforts: We want our worth back.

Food has power over you because of weight stigmas you get from society, and it triggers a lack of self-acceptance in you. It's been said many times that there is connection between food and mood and that how we eat can influence blood sugar, cravings, and energy throughout the day. I believe we don't talk about the mood and food connection enough. Mood eating, compulsive eating behaviors, and struggling for a perfect body, happens as we play out our insecurities in them and strive for worthiness.

It's like society says there are prerequisites for worthiness, and if you don't have the body you envisioned, you are not quite worthy of love and belonging. This is why we spend years if not decades of time and effort to attain the perfect body we wish to have.

You use your body shape and weight as a measuring stick for your self-worth and personal value. What others say and think about your body is more important than how you feel. You believe that if you are approved externally from others as good enough regarding your shape, you will be liked more, and in the meantime you will develop more self-worth and self-love.

On one side of the coin, you have body-image insecurity and a lack of self-worth and self-love. On the other side, you want to have a happy life. These two are tightly related to each other and connected to limiting beliefs about yourself. The media does put some effort into supporting women to love their bodies in any shape and form. However, the problem is that the media at large does not look at the underlying cause of body-image insecurity. Although body-image campaigns tell you that you can be beautiful in any shape and size—and this is something great—they don't work as well as we would like them to. This is because the self-image, self-acceptance, and inherent worth of the girls and woman who see these campaigns are already attached to one thought: "I am not good enough because I am not thin enough." Or they think, "Having a job I want, a boyfriend I want, friends I want, and ultimately the life I want can't happen because I don't look thin enough, so I am not good enough." Girls and woman hold themselves back because they think that to get what they want, they first need to get thin.

Since when do we translate being thin enough to mean being good enough?

I can't tell you I have no idea why you feel this way, because I was there for a long time. I attached my worth to the number on the scale or the size of the pants I wore. I noticed that although I lost weight a lot of times, how I felt toward myself didn't change much. I was pushing myself with chronic dieting and exercising, and I hated every day when I wasn't eating right or skipped exercising. It was a very bad place to be. But even though I was thin for a while, I was emotionally unstable, feeling lots of fear and unworthiness. My life was a constant battle to feel I was good enough.

Whenever we compare ourselves with others, judge ourselves, beat ourselves up, or belittle ourselves, we ignore our magnificence and walk away from our values and our sense of worth. You don't need to be fixed. You are enough the way you are. But until you believe it, no one will. We each have something unique to give to the world, and that gives us worth. Our birthright is being worthy, no matter what. The idea that we don't deserve our worth is a collective human disorder. Of course, just by looking around, we constantly hear and see advertisements and marketing campaigns about what we need to buy to become worthy. We are so brainwashed at so many levels that we basically develop subconscious self-hate. Self-worth is such a basic human thing to possess. It shouldn't even be a question. When did we start to lose it?

The icing on the cake is that chronic dieting and emotional eating is not really about food, as we've discussed. Similarly, body-image insecurity and body shame is not really about your body. They are both about the lack of feeling worthy of love.

If you are in an ongoing battle with weight fluctuation and you go on diets again and again to look better and feel better about yourself, reaching your goal weight won't fill up the empty place inside of you— the idea that you are not enough. It's not victim mentality but total powerlessness. The feeling of not being enough is like an invisible handicap from a lack of self-acceptance and often self-hate. So, you turn to food to fill up that emptiness inside.

If you can't or don't change the way you think about yourself, and if you don't feel loved inside because you are unable to love yourself, you will never be truly happy. If you can't feel a sense of self-worth and self-love, you won't be able to take care of yourself when your emotional needs need to be met. Eventually, no matter what problem you might have, whether it's related to a relationship, job, or weight issues, all challenges stems from a lack of self-love.

When our only purpose with weight management is external, we may never find real happiness. If we seek happiness in our looks, activities, or vocation, we are setting ourselves up for failure. When we lose a job or the appearance we like, it feels like losing ourselves. Therefore, if you are working on losing weight or maintaining it but don't change how you talk to yourself and feel about yourself, the weight will come back eventually.

This is true even if you get more love from people around you. If you are not able to love and respect yourself, no amount of affection from others can make up for it. Knowing yourself and why you do the things you do is great, but it is even more important to live from a place of loving yourself.

This is worth repeating: The real issue is that no matter how much love you get from people for being slim, it is going to be difficult for you to manage your weight if the thinness doesn't come from having a sense of self-worth, self-love, and emotional balance. If you are only rigidly focused on a diet and exercise regimen, pushing aside feelings to impress yourself and others as you strive to be liked more, most likely your weight will fluctuate all the time.

In other words, if you manage to lose weight or stay at your goal weight by hating your body and pushing, restricting, or controlling it, you will still hate it at your ideal weight.

I am sure you've experienced this when you were at your ideal weight or very close to your happy weight at some point in your life; you knew you were supposed to be happy, but you weren't. This is because you chose to lose weight by hating your body constantly. Why would you have a different feeling at the end? If we continue managing our weight by hating our bodies, we will stay miserable for the rest of our lives and constantly try to be in control. Or, more often than not, we will keep losing and gaining the weight all the time in a diet-binge cycle.

I hear from women and girls regularly that they just can't accept or don't want to accept their bodies. They believe that if they accept it, it will never change.

I can absolutely understand why someone would feel like this, but let's ask a different question. If hating or refusing to accept your body and constantly judging and criticizing it worked, almost every woman on earth would be thin already and at peace with her body. Similarly, if the way we approach dieting worked in the long run, we would all be permanently thin.

The real work is to finally realize that the only reason we are so addicted to our look and shape is that we not only want to look good but also feel good enough.

You might ask, "How can we pinpoint and address the insecurities that keep me thinking I am not good enough or I am not worthy of love and belonging? How do I get to the point when I trust myself with food and I know what's best for me?"

The whole point of this book is not about getting you to a place where you trust yourself with food. It's about getting you to a place where you can trust *yourself*. When you can feel at peace with yourself, you will feel at peace around food as well because they are the same thing.

For you, food is what you use and what you have made special to anesthetize your discomfort. So, how do you get to a place where you feel comfortable with food? Let's instead ask the following: How do you get to a place where you feel comfortable with yourself? By being comfortable with yourself, your relationship to food will change. That's why self-acceptance and loving yourself is so important.

When you are able to change your perception and your beliefs and you truly live from a place of self-worth and self-love, your actions will change eventually, leading exactly in the direction you want to go. When we move toward the intent to learn, one of the things we must learn about is who we really are.

> **Fighting For A Perfect, Thin Body = Fighting For Worthiness**
> **Since When Thin Enough = Good Enough?**

Chronic Dieting And Emotional Eating Is Not Really About Food
Body Image Insecurity And Body Shame Is Not Really About Your Body
They Are Both About The Lack Of Self-Worth, The Lack Of Feeling Worthy Of Love
And The Lack Of Feeling Deserving To Be Loved

True Happiness Doesn't Lie In A Perfect Body
True Happiness = It's In the Ability Of Loving Yourself And Feeling A Sense Of Self-Worth
No Matter What Other People Think Of You

No Amount Of Love From Others Can Diminish Your Suffering.
Although We All Love To Be Cherished And Worshiped By Others,
If You Can't Love And Appreciate Yourself, Your Happiness Will Be Always
Based On What People Think Of You And How They Treat You

To Overcome The Struggle Of Permanent Weight Loss Is Not
About Getting You A Place Where You Can Trust Yourself With Food.
It is About Getting You A Place Where You Can Trust Yourself.

When You Feel At Peace With Yourself = You Will Feel At Peace Around Food
Because They Are The Same Thing

Your Inner Critic

If you were not allowed or encouraged to express yourself in childhood, you might still believe that it is inappropriate to do so. If your caregivers were judgmental toward you as you grew up, most likely you developed a sense of loneliness and feeling unworthy. It is probably hard for you to ask for what you need or stand up for yourself.

There are many people who grew up in self-nurturing environments and still feel like they have an inner critic who is always judgmental, negative, and shaming. In fact, we all have an inner critic. But not all of us react to the point where it gets in the way of living a full life.

Among girls and women, negative self-talk creates invisible handicaps. I wouldn't have to be a nutritionist to know how much girls and women are concerned with being skinny enough or pretty enough to be liked and accepted.

The inner critic consumes our lives big time. This source of negative self-talk holds us back from who we actually are, and this drives our eating habits as well. Can you imagine all the gifts and talents we could give to the world? But without self-worth and self-acceptance, we are not able to bring these gifts to the surface. How many of us live small lives because of this negative self-talk? I realized self-rejection is the primary reason we have this huge epidemic of yo-yo dieters and struggles with weight.

Your willingness to go on diets over and over again, eat emotionally, and have the goal of fixing your body must benefit you somehow; otherwise, you wouldn't do it.

However, as mentioned previously, issues around eating are inevitably connected to issues of love. They indicate issues with lack of self-love, lack of self-worth, lack of self-acceptance, self-rejection, self-denial, or power. These feelings are all connected to food issues, as they are all tools for you to fill or control an inner emptiness.

Remember the following perspective:

Food is not the enemy.
Your life is not the enemy.
People are not your enemy.
Self-hate is your enemy.
It's time to love yourself first!

It is important that you know yourself and know your goals and values in life, but how you treat yourself in the meantime is the most significant thing.

Self-Worth

When you believe that body shape or beauty attracts happiness and love and of you think that you are not beautiful, you declare that you are not worthy of love and happiness. Having a low level of confidence in your body and believing that you are only worthy of love or happiness of your body is in great shape, you will reject the love and affection all around you. You will not even notice it.

Losing Self-Worth from the Media

In our society, it is common to control our weight by restricting what we eat. By doing this, we declare that there must be something wrong with us if we are overweight, and we deserve body stigma for not taking care of ourselves. The media and social and cultural expectations cause us to lose self-worth, and we struggle with body-image insecurity. Do you watch TV, read magazines, or listen to the radio? Feeling shame about your body can be traced back to larger social expectations like families of origin and cultural messages, including those from the media and stereotypes. We have all felt the pain wash over us when we feel stared at, judged, or teased about the way we look. Sometimes, someone else puts us down or ridicules us, but more often, we are hard on ourselves in the form of negative self-talk. The never-ending fight to feel worthy and accepted is relentless.

We are bombarded with media-driven messages about so-called normalcy. We want to know what's normal because we think it affords" us a greater opportunity for acceptance and belonging.

Many advertisements, however, prey on the vulnerabilities of women by exploiting their need to feel normal. When we are easily influenced, we are more likely to reinforce the messages we see and hear. We individualize the problems and feel like our inability to meet the social expectations is because of our own deficiencies or pathologies.

In regard to appearance and body image, it's not the quest for perfection that is so painful. Failing to meet the unattainable expectations is what leads to the painful feeling of shame washing over us.

With the lack of positive self-concept and a lack of understanding who we are, we are all headed toward the unfair expectations driven by the media, almost by default.

Psychologically speaking, we are taking our cues for body-image satisfaction from certain environments, such as family, friends, and our social and cultural background as well as from the media we are surrounded with. Based on these cues, we have certain expectations of how we are supposed to look, and if we don't, we create imaginary flaws.

These expectations and unrealistic cultural standards are easily translated into feelings of not being good enough. All we've ever known is to accept the standards that life puts on us instead of realizing them as unrealistic expectations. So in the absence of critical awareness and self-care skills, we lose our self-acceptance and start to compensate for a lack of self-worth by controlling our appetites and bodies.

Sometimes, it doesn't matter how much your caregivers told you that you were loved and that your body was beautiful as you grew up. You have little control over media influences. There is a saying, "Keeping people safe from the media culture is like asking them not to breath to keep them safe from air pollution." It soaks into our DNA; the media becomes part of who we are. Unfortunately, not having the perfect body is a huge shame trigger for most women.

Our brains are pretty much genetically trained to believe what our eyes see. We are extremely influenced by advertising. The lifestyles ads sell tell us what we need to have, be, or do to obtain worth, love, sexuality, popularity, and normalcy. According to Jean Kilbourne, internationally recognized for her work about how media images influence our life, says that we are each exposed to over three thousand ads a day. Therefore, how we feel about ourselves and what we desire is extremely influenced by advertising. And yet, remarkably, most of us believe that we are not. Ads sell a great deal more than products. They sell values, images, and concepts. They tell us who we are and who we should be. Sometimes they sell addictions. Although ads may seem harmless and silly, they add up to a powerful form of cultural conditioning.

Marketing is used to make a product or service irresistible, making us feel that our life can't be complete without the product or service in question. But marketing is basically applied psychology, where experts understand how to connect the heart, brain, and emotions to make you feel like you must get or achieve what they say to be happy and successful.

You may still wonder why we feel like crap most of the time. It's because all these advertisements are sending messages something like the following: If you look perfect and do everything perfectly, keeping a smile on your face, you will be appreciated and admired, and you will reach happiness. Doesn't just reading it feel exhausting? These are the expectations we all try to meet. We all tend to see our flaws rather than the beauty inside of us. Every culture impacted by the Western media has this phenomenon. Body dysmorphia and body-image dissatisfaction is a huge issue all over the world.

We shouldn't be surprised if we are looking for something to munch on when the expectations are so high that our emotional resources are drained. We hear from the media that happiness is in our clothes, shoes, and sunglasses. We never hear, "You can find happiness in how you treat yourself, living in harmony with inner peace sensation. We hear that what you look like is more important than who you are. And you end up thinking that if you don't meet those criteria, you should feel flawed and unworthy.

Losing Self-Worth from Family of Origin

Our identity become influenced by our family of origin, such as its geographic makeup, nationality, or the family system we were born into. Childhood is the stage of your life when you go with the flow and do not have many philosophical ideas about your surroundings or the way you live. You are willing to learn almost anything that comes across your path. You can see this if you watch a child grow through all the different phases of understanding as he or she begins to walk, talk, and communicate. The evolution of your psychological development happens when you are between eighteen and forty-two months old; this is when you develop your autonomy.

At this age, we start to develop a sense of self—what we want and don't want and what we will or won't do. In the meantime, our caregivers teach us how to behave, and we model our thinking to fit into society without even knowing it. As a child, you establish your independence at some point. This is the realization of separateness, when you internalize an understanding that you are separate from your caregivers and your environment, and you have the right to ask things and to have free will as an individual.

If you look at a child at this age, you can notice how he or she works out this autonomy. The young person builds boundaries unconsciously, feeling out what works for you and what doesn't.

When you get to your adolescent stage, you try to establish your autonomy again and convey your true sense of how you see the world. As we become more communicative and mobile, we get new sets of rules about the proper way to get around in this world. You follow all the rules and requests by default most of the time. Your family and teachers show you how to behave appropriately in society. When you are a child, you don't get to choose your own belief system. It is all there, handed to you the moment you are born. Parents and caregivers model a way of living and thinking by expecting certain behaviors, and then they reward or punish you based on how you perform. Your parents, friends, and people around you were also trained by rewards and punishments. This is the cycle of life.

During childhood, you were dependent on your family. When your caregivers provide you with self-nurturing behaviors, you can develop skills that help you understand, handle, and express emotions. Were your caregivers kind, empathic, patient, and comforting? Did they let you have personal boundaries? Did they give you reasonable limits, treat you fairly, respect you, and make you feel loved and valued? Or did you grow up with critical, negative, judgmental, obsessive, fearful thoughts, feeling insecure, unsafe, and abused verbally or physically?

Most of us grew up with mothers and fathers who used harsh criticism to keep us out of trouble. When you're growing up, you hear things like, "Don't do that … just because I said so," "shame on you," "you are a bad girl," or "you are stupid." As a child, you understand that if you are not playing by the book, you get into trouble.

Although punishment is directed to producing good behavior, it usually goes deeper than that, unfortunately. We tend to internalize the judgmental, critical, unkind, or shaming voice of our caregivers and let it repeat inside our head. Although you might think you don't deserve to be treated certain ways, you may assume that criticism is good and necessary so that when you grow up, you can be critical toward yourself as well to fit in.

As a child, you believe that you must go through these socialization patterns; otherwise, you wouldn't be experiencing them. This method of parenting give you a sense of worth from being good, and a lack of self-worth can came from being bad. Human nature is like that. Based on what you hear, you make the assumption that something is wrong with you sometimes. That's why you get punished. It isn't even a conscious thought process; you just assume certain behaviors are what good people do.

The world around you works so that you think you deserve to suffer when you are bad, and you don't deserve to be happy unless you are good. You may also think you don't deserve to be loved if you are bad. Therefore, you make the assumption that you need to be good in order to be loved, and you must be bad when you don't get the love you want. What we internalize at early age can have a huge impact on our adult life. Self-defeating thoughts can result in frustration, avoidance, procrastination, people-pleasing, or striving for perfection to cope with unpleasant emotions and thoughts.

If you find yourself in situations where you can't express what you want or when your needs don't get met, you can lose your ground instead of freely expressing your will or accepting the situation.

But I am not here to attack your parents or caregivers. They also come from a set of behavioral patterns presented to them when they were young. They learned how to behave in society just like you—what to believe and what not to, what is acceptable and what is not, what is good and what is bad, what is beautiful and what is ugly, and what is right and what is wrong. That knowledge and those rules and concepts about how to behave were there at their birth. And you not only rely on people around you but also believe the mirror that they show you about who you are. Therefore, your understanding about how loveable you are is based on how people treat you.

The conditioning from our individual household can lead to certain thinking and behavioral patterns within us. It can help to form a nurturing and loving relationship with ourselves, but it can also create a negative or mean girl inside of us.

If we grow up with skills that represent our true being, we develop a balanced true self and can have warm, loving, and kind relationships with ourselves. Some of these traits include being responsible and reliable, setting effective boundaries, having a sense of humor with the world and with ourselves, having high self-esteem, being able to meet challenges in life, practicing self-acceptance, being spontaneous, and having a sense of self-worth, and having a carefree relationship with ourselves.

But none come from a perfect family, where all our needs were met exactly the way we wanted. If we don't have self-nurturing skills intuitively or based on examples, we can wind up having a pretty bad relationship with ourselves.

Evaluate your life for a moment to see how easy it is for you to take action freely and how easily you express what you need or want. Who are the people that trigger you, and you go along with what they want. Is it hard for you speak your truth in your career? We start to lose our sense of self when we repress a certain part of ourselves or deny what's important to us.

Psychologist Dr. Margaret Paul explains that a big part of our psychological health is seated in our upbringing. If we felt rejected and misunderstood or if our caregivers were not emotionally available, we develop a sense of shame. She calls it the "core shame," and it comes from the false belief that there is something intrinsically wrong with us—we are inherently bad, wrong, defective, flawed, unimportant, unworthy, or inadequate. As small children, if we didn't get the love we needed, we may have concluded that it was our fault rather than our parents' inability to love us in a way we needed to be loved. Because we believed this, we constantly tried to look right and perform right to get others to like us, love us, or approve of us. We felt worthy only when we were receiving validation from others.

We thought that if we didn't get the validation, we must not deserve it. The only way we could feel a sense of control was from believing that the behavior of others was our fault. We concluded that since their lack of love was our fault, we must have been somehow defective. We also believed that we could have control over how others saw us and felt about us. Therefore, if someone didn't like us, it must be our fault: "Did I say something wrong?" "What did I do wrong?" we wondered. By believing it is our fault, we felt a sense of control. We concluded, "If it is my fault that someone doesn't like me, I just have to figure out how to do it right, and then I can control how others feel about me."

If we had recognized our parents' wounds and limitations, we would have felt crushingly helpless about getting the love we needed. Instead, most of us chose to try to have control over getting the love we needed and over avoiding the rejection or abuse we feared.

We feel unsafe, sometimes consciously, when our whole sense of worth hinges upon having control over getting others' approval. We may feel panicked when we fear making mistakes and risking disapproval and rejection. We may judge ourselves in our effort to look right or do things the right way. We all have core beliefs from our childhood that still operate on autopilot—we continue to act out of them whether we realize it or not.

A core belief can be an assumed truth or assumed reality, based on what you see, hear, and think about situations via your lenses—the way you see the world. There is no one lens. We all have our own individual perspective. We each come from different backgrounds, and we each absorb and understand the world based on our own perception.

Interestingly enough, we are all looking for the same thing: love, joy, and happiness.

Even though core beliefs are unconscious, they are backed up with confidence, faith, trust, and acceptance. The problem is that we forget that we actually chose to believe in our core shame. Many of us now operate out of it as if it is our identity.

Julie M. Simson, a psychotherapist who specializes in overeaters, writes the following in her book *The Emotional Eater's Repair Manual* about what our caregivers model: "It's important that our caregivers model positive, hopeful thinking and help us replace any pessimistic, self-doubting, or fearful thoughts. It's helpful when caregivers regularly express joy, happiness, and even excitement so we know that these emotional states are also possible and acceptable."

She continues saying that when our caregivers allow us free emotional expression and help us meet our needs, we learn to trust our signals and the goodwill of others. In this loving atmosphere, we develop an inner sense of safety, security, and trust as well as a feeling of worthiness. We naturally develop self-acceptance and self-love. We learn where we end and the world begins and that it's okay to have personal boundaries. We learn that there will always be enough. We also learn how to set reasonable limits and delay gratification of our impulses so that we can take the best care of ourselves and meet personal goals. The kindness and goodwill of our caregivers foster the formation of a solid sense of self and good self-esteem. We establish our unique identity as our caregivers encourage our growing autonomy. Additionally, we are able to separate from them, having developed a capacity for intimacy and love of ourselves and others. Personal boundaries are a sort of invisible psychological edge that defines where we end and another person, or the world, begins. When our caregivers model firm-yet-flexible healthy boundaries, we grow up with clear, healthy boundaries of our own. If your boundaries tend to be too loose, you'll become merged or enmeshed with others and their needs. You may have difficulty identifying and expressing your own needs and asking for support in meeting them.

The society we live in is not particularly a model of self-nurturing skills. You might have grown up in an environment where, for a variety of reasons, your basic physical and emotional needs were inadequately met. Perhaps insecurity is all you ever knew. In your childhood, you may have had to maintain your guard against emotional or physical abuse. Emotional negligence can be felt as trauma in the form of abandonment, attack, betrayal, blame, neglect, rejection, or shame.

Trauma results in and forces us to cope with chronic unpleasant emotional states, such as anxiety, depression, sadness, emptiness, hurt, loneliness, and guilt.

Most of us don't develop self-nurturing skills to check expectations against reality and protect ourselves from unwanted identities. As an adult, your job is to understand that if you have a tendency to let other people tell you how smart you are, your whole self-worth will depend on those opinions. None of us comes from a perfectly capable household. You can't expect to be taught what self-worth is, especially if you were raised by adults who had no idea what it was themselves.

But you are not a child anymore. You can take care of yourself. When you believe you are inherently defective and that you have to hide your true self to be acceptable, that's when your wounded self takes over and loses touch with your core self—who you really are. If, for example, you are stuck defining yourself through your look and performance, you are suffering the anxiety that comes from being vulnerable to others' disapproval." Are you willing to do the work that needs to be done in order to remember your self-worth and to feel, act, and live accordingly?

Everything in this chapter regarding how you think related to your self-worth and body image can be used as a huge wake-up call. Going forward, I would like you to understand that if judgment regarding your body shape, weight, or size gets to you, then it is not what it is said about you that makes you feel hurt. What hurts is that you let the words tear you down. Even before they were spoken, deep down, you believed in them.

Letting go of negative comments and feelings from others about your body and meeting your own needs and desires can lead you toward happiness and confidence with your body. If you believe that no one will love you or find you sexy because you are too short, tall, or fat, then you are heading to a dead end. Your weight-loss journey has to be about you, not what your significant other or society wants from you. If you do it for others, it will be a willpower game eventually. If it comes from within you, it will be from a loving place instead of fear. This is not only sustainable but also it feels so good. It is not about pushing or restricting yourself anymore but allowing and surrendering what you want and what feels good to you.

Part III
Making the Jump

"It takes courage to grow up and be who you really are."
—E.E. Cummings

How To Transform Your Body Through the Way You See Things

The only thing I can tell you at this stage is that your life has its own way to let you know what is truly happening in your life. You need to shift or remembers something to feel joyful and fulfilled and get the body that you want so desperately.

Permanent weight loss is not just about what you put on your plate. It's also about how you feel about what you eat and how you treat yourself.

If you are reading this book, I will assume that you are open to a more holistic and feminine approach when it comes to permanent weight loss. Mainstream weight loss practices emphasize pushing, controlling, and limiting yourself, which is a very masculine approach. I will be approaching weight and food issues from a more feminine and permissive perspective. This approach goes beyond nutrition and exercise, combining science, self-care, personal growth, and psychology to bring permanent weight loss.

When you add more life-affirming principles, it will result in success. We have all learned from an early age that to get or achieve something, we need to fight for it. We learned that if we don't like something about ourselves, accepting it or surrendering to it means we will never change, and we will be stuck with our flaws forever. When we don't like our body, we almost want to hammer it out by hating it and restricting it with nutrition and guilt-ridden exercise. But what really shapes the body is inner peace. Our ability (or inability) to accept ourselves it what keeps us stuck in one place. We are so focused on fighting what we don't want that we don't even realize that the act of laser focus on something we don't want, and we try to ignore what gives power to the very thing we don't want in control. Ongoing weight struggles, chronic dieting, and being in an unhappy place with your body are more than a food issue; it is an emotional issue.

Years of going on and off of calorie restrictions, diets, and obsession with weight, size, and body image is disguised as a path to happiness in mind. However, I am sure you realize by now how easy it is to fall prey to quick, easy, or long-term promises. You probably know deep down that it is not quite working for you, even though there is always a new and better way to manage your weight in the diet industry and in the media. Quick fixes might even be working for you in a short period of time, but long-term success is nowhere to be found. Why is that?

You can have a naturally thin body without pushing and controlling, but you need a new approach. Until you let go of the limitations you have created around restrictive dieting or compulsive eating, you can't see what motivates you to create them. Permanent weight loss is first a self-love issue and not a food issue.

If you seek to move past all of the issues with chronic dieting, body-image insecurity, or emotional eating, you need to understand your attachment to them. Instead of focusing on external tools as you might be doing with nutrition and exercise, you have to be willing to do the time-consuming, deep, honest inner work that brings real transformation.

Behind diets, there are the habits of restricting and overeating, which come from trying to get control over your body to be liked and loveable. Behind emotional eating, you may have feelings of insecurity or uncertainty that manifest as an imbalanced emotional state. But behind all of these things, you're pursuing a feeling of worthiness, as discussed previously. Food is a means to get the love you crave. It numbs the pain inside, alters consciousness, and fills up your inner emptiness. Food provides a sense of security and enjoyment that is far easier to deal with than the pain. By not feeling the discomfort, you can maintain an illusion of happiness.

As a holistic health practitioner, I truly believe that although nutrition and exercise are important factors in weight management, focusing solely on them cannot provide the peace with food to stop chronic dieting or emotional eating. You can't really have a healthy, lean appearance and feel peace inside without being connected to all four pillars (physical, emotional, mental, and spiritual), especially if you are a chronic dieter, if you use food as a copying mechanism, or if you have body-image insecurity.

The key to releasing your excess weight and staying lean is multidimensional. The behavioral, emotional, nutritional, and metabolic issues all need to be addressed. You must work through the pillars and do all the recommended introspection to achieve a stable body weight. When you do that, you will feel a deep sense of personal fulfillment, and this is ultimately what you are after, so it is a win-win situation.

Your unique challenge in permanent weight-loss resistance might be any of the following:

- Dieting triggers the diet-binge cycle because of restrictions
- You might be missing key nutrients from food, making you hungry all the time
- Whether you eat healthy or unhealthy, unstable blood sugar might make you feel weak and have low energy—hence the desire to eat constantly all day long
- Emotional eating habits
- Body-image insecurity and body shame make you crazy around food

If you are able to get in touch with your real desire (and you will), your body will manifest in its leanest form from within. You will perhaps have to face some of your demons or limiting beliefs, but if you can, self-acceptance, self-love, and feeling worthy is waiting for you along with your healthy, lean body.

Many of us who struggle with dieting, emotional eating, or body image fail to hear the sweetness of our own song because we are too busy listening to the voice of others, whether it is our caregivers, friends, classmates, teachers, husband, colleagues, or the culture we live in. Instead of listening to our own voice and expressing who we are, we let others define what our needs are, what we should do, how we should look, and what standards we should live by. We can feel responsible to keep the family, friendships, and work relationships together and forget about our needs.

We sacrifice our desires and fix what's wrong in an effort to make everything all right. Since we can't even hear our voice—our desires—and we can't connect with ourselves, we live to eat as a source of pleasure and comfort instead of eating to live. That's what is causing some of your problems. We must stop sacrificing our needs, even when others insist we should be silent. We must recognize our need for me time—a period set aside for reflection to listen to your voice. Through this voice, we can get in touch with our feelings and give ourselves the chance to get nourished. Our feelings can help us find the balance between our relationship with ourselves and our relationship with others. Finding and listening to our own voice, the expression of our true sense of self, can nourish us and free us from eating out of emotions.

I stated at the beginning of the book that the reasons you have weight struggles is because you diet, you eat less and exercise more, you eat emotionally, or you are trapped in body shame, but I believe you are ready to hear that none of these is the actual reason for your weight struggle. These are only the effects of the real reasons that hide behind these activities.

We are meant to discover the real issues and release the needs that cause excess weight, chronic dieting, body shame, and more. Regardless of what kind of unwanted identities you picked up along the way during your childhood, your cultural environment, and from the media, your peace of mind now depends on circumstances. If feelings of stress, anxiety, or boredom compel you to eat, you might be missing the outlets where you can convey and move through those emotions. By being aware of what's truly going on in your life and addressing those needs, you will be successful at managing your weight and eating patterns.

Your success will be firmly based on the work you have done on yourself from the inside out. The external world will start to match your internal world, not the other way around. Most of us think that when our external world looks a certain way—for example, when we are at the size we are supposed to be, the inside will get better. But in the long run, you can't win with this attitude. However, if you are truly aware of your needs, understand them, and are able to meet them—including your emotional needs—the external world will follow, and you will get the body you want effortlessly. On the other hand, as mentioned previously, exercising, dieting, and covering up emotions with food are all the result of an internal problem.

If you want to have a long-lasting change physically, it needs to start with accepting where you are right now. Accept the fact that you don't need to be fixed. There is nothing wrong with you. If you can embrace self-acceptance wherever you are in your life journey right now and be open about your struggles, then you can start your self-improvement journey despite any struggles that come your way.

Additionally, people who eat emotionally—maybe just like you—while overeating or body-image insecurities might not be a real issue, but they tend to numb their feelings with food for the sake of mental and emotional nourishment.

Diets directly correlate to our body-image insecurities. Emotional eating can occur for cognitive issues, which relate to body shame, but there can be plenty of people who binge or eat emotionally without a direct correlation to body shame or lack of body acceptance. In this case, it is a compulsive behavior around food to check out from their problems or emotions, which could be related to anything but body issues.

Most of the time, emotional eating is not caused by body-image insecurity and a lack of accepting your body, but it can cause you to have them. Emotional eaters gain weight eventually, and body issues come up a lot of the time.

Eating to numb your feelings or to ignore your physical hunger can often be seen as two different things, but they are not. Both are the result of you disconnecting from your body so that you don't have to feel. Being aware of what limiting beliefs make you do such things can be an eye opener and a huge gift. You can't change what you don't know.

When you are using food out of real hunger or simply for enjoyment, without feeling guilty or ashamed, food serves its purpose. But when you restrict your food, overeat, or any other emotional eating behaviors we've discussed, food is filling a need as a counterfeit. It can be used for multiple reasons, which might seem like a short-term course of action, but when you do it over an extended period of time, weight gain appears as a physical sign.

Although body-image insecurities are prevalent among women and girls who diet and not necessarily among those who eat emotionally, in both categories, people are hurting their body by not honoring its hunger and satiety signals. There is a lack of love for their bodies. To routinely overlook your body's needs, you must be detached or feel separated from your body—regardless of the reasons. In other words, no matter why you engage in emotional eating (a mental, emotional, or spiritual disconnection) or riding the diet-binge cycle, at the end of the day, you are dishonoring your body, which is ultimately a reflection of your lack of self-love and self-acceptance.

However, by respecting your body's hunger and satiety (the need for rest, movement, etc.) you will create a bridge to reconnect with your body. Once you do this, you will be able to feel connection, compassion, and self-acceptance for your body. And then all the issues you have stuffed down with food start to come to the surface; this can be the gateway to find a permanent solution for your weight struggle.

It is in eye-opening, beautiful, and challenging process—an amazing healing journey. It is about turning your challenges and wounds into wisdom. Chronic dieting, emotional eating, body-image insecurity, and weight struggle is so much more than what you thought it was. I hope you realize this by now. When you try to untangle, be aware that you can not only let go of what you've been stuffing down but also remember who you are and be a new you.

One of the underlying causes of ongoing weight fluctuations and on-and-off dieting for years if not decades lies in body-image insecurity. This is the driving force of our willingness to deprive ourselves on diets that lead to binges. Not everybody who is a compulsive eater struggles with weight issues and body shame. But in the end, *the diet mentality and emotional eating are both caused by disowning our bodies because we use it as a punching bag to avoid crappy feelings.* Using willpower for dieting is as difficult on the mind in the long run as feeling disconnected, feeling insecure, or having a scarcity mind-set when you feel happy or excited about something. So we instead anesthetize the feelings we don't want to feel or don't know how to handle.

In order to have a great relationship with your body, with yourself, and with your life, you need to understand that the physical condition you experience (weight fluctuation, compulsive behavior toward food, body hate, or insecurity) is directly connected to your connection to life, your beliefs, and your emotional state. Before you can manage either your weight or emotional eating, you need to find and heal the root cause of your beliefs and feelings. Only then you can achieve lasting results with your issues.

Instead of looking at your struggle as a burden, be willing to see your physical or emotional issues as a means to discover who you are when all the pretenses are stripped away. Most of the time, we only get down on our knees and look for solutions beyond nutrition and exercise when we hit rock bottom. After years of trial and error, we get tired of dealing with all the craziness around food and body.

My personal struggle with weight, food, and emotional imbalances started with influences from different directions. There was a lot of anxiety around food while I was growing up. Although our family meals were scheduled, and it seemed normal, it was hectic when the family gathered around the table, and somehow I experienced a lot of anxiety around food. I picked up my weight stigmas from being a dancer and from working in the TV business for so long, where looks were really important. Soothing myself with food was not something I consciously chose, but it became second nature over time. With nutrition and exercise, I was able to manage my weight more or less, but peace around food and my body was nowhere to be found. I could only let go of craziness around food and my obsession with weight when I was willing to dig deeper and look behind the underlying reasons for my weight fluctuations and compulsive eating.

Looking back, where I was then and where I am now is very different. I am now at peace around food and with my body because all the issues that I had rose to the surface in my life. Those issues were the source of the nagging feeling I had of not being good enough. Although I have been successful many areas of my life, the toxic habits led me down a path of having the willingness to heal my body and mind. I had to feel my emotions and believe in what made me who I was, not what I was expected to become.

When you can really grasp of the idea that your body is only the expression of how you think and the result of what you do, you will subconsciously choose better thoughts. You will also have better feelings as you respect of the truth of who you are instead of abusing yourself with food, thoughts, or relationships. Changing your body starts with focusing on the right mind-set, but first and foremost, a shift in perception is needed, wherein you believe that the ultimate purpose of your body is to express how you feel and go in the direction of love instead of fear. If you want to be loved or respected, first you have to respect your body. It's like the relationship you have toward your life is mirrored by the relationship you have with your body. If your life is hectic, your eating will be hectic, and the relationship you have with yourself will be hectic. If you want nurturing relationships in your life, first and foremost, you have to be able to nurture yourself. The same thing goes with how you want to feel in your life. You can't want abundance; you have to feel it first. You have to feel and believe in happiness before you get it.

When you can find the catalyst that changes you so there is no more emotional eating, weight fluctuation, or body-image insecurity, that's the point where you can have and will have a fit body and a healthy relationship with food and your body. Said another way, when your body's weight stops fluctuating and you can easily manage your weight or stop emotional eating, it will be the result of getting rid of all your mental or emotional crap.

To obtain permanent weight loss, holistic nutrition is the key to finding the answers via the physical, emotional, mental, and spiritual aspects:

- The issue can be physically driven. Your body craves essential nutrients from food in order to function properly, and this triggers the feeling of hunger.
- The issue can be related to an emotional appetite to fill up a hole inside.
- The issue can be low self-worth and poor self-love that manifest in bad body image and negative thoughts about the self.
- The issue can be emptiness in the soul, with feelings of disconnection and purposelessness.

Establish Self-Care Skills

Compulsive eating has its own pain, and labeling compulsive eating the bad guy just creates shame and guilt associated with the act, which is not something I support. Therefore, we should not look at this activity as a bad thing. Trying to avoid something we've categorized as bad makes it hard to see what it is actually we are trying to avoid. Looking under the hood to find the trigger points and to engage your true appetite is the solution.

Emotional eating shouldn't lead you to beat yourself up for eating what you are not supposed to; it should cause you to dig deeper and discover what you are looking for in that food. Creating rules around emotional eating without looking at the emotional drive—the reason for the urge to eat—will not lead to feel relaxed around food and only adds to the problem.

When you get into the habit of self-care and self-connection, the desire to eat emotionally can be seen as an alarm that goes off in your mind as a clue that something bothers you, and you need to deal with it.

I invite you to think about food as your friend, not as your enemy. You will only protect yourself with food when you feel the need or desire to eat without being physically hungry, so food is really a guardian angel to remind you that you need to take care of something you feel.

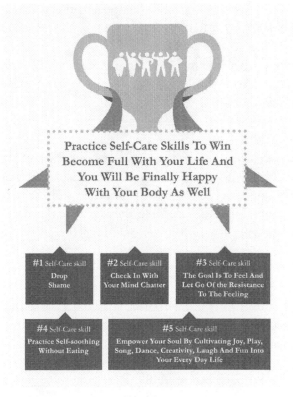

Self-Care Skill One: Drop Shame

Eating healthy most of the time is important for staying healthy in the long run and for having good energy throughout the day. But when you have a compulsive behavior around food, caring how you feel about what you put in your mouth is as important as how healthy your eating habits are. Sometimes, people feel that eating fast or watching TV while eating is necessary because they want to avoid being present with the food. This is because being present with food means being present with guilt, shame, and negative self-talk.

By dropping shame around the so-called mistakes that you make when you diet, eat emotionally, or feel body shame, we can start untangling all the things behind the feeling and understand the root cause of your weight struggle.

Why Dropping Shame Is Crucial for Your Success

Women and girls just like you have a lot of shame and fear-based thoughts about who they are and what they are worth. As I described in preceding chapters, we diet, eat emotionally, and have body-image insecurity because we are fighting for our worth.

We are ashamed of who we are because that's what society and media tell us to feel. Your environment can make you believe that you are not good enough the way you are. When you can't identify your core values, you will get lost between social ideals and your own core values. And the moment that you believe you are not enough, unworthiness can hold you hostage and impact your life because you subconsciously carry the story of your shame. Shame tells you that you are not good enough. *But your net worth has nothing to do with your self-worth.* I like to remind myself of this. Society likes to define us by how much we make, what we possess, and what we do for living. We naturally place so much value on these things, and then we wonder why it is so hard to separate our identities from them.

Shame keeps us small; we want to hide and punish ourselves. We don't want to be judged by others. Many times we subconsciously accumulate body weight, hoping to get some protection from the outside world. Emotional weight is something a lot of women experience. Releasing the pain can lead to releasing the excess weight as well.

How Shame Is Applied in Your Struggle

A feeling of shame is pervasive among women and girls. Beauty standards are high, and we live in a society where it is a standard cultural expectation to do everything perfectly without showing the effort behind it. I touched on this briefly in a previous chapter.

If you look back in time, you might be able to trace back to a point in your life when you got your first shame triggers around your body; sometimes they are less obvious. You might remember someone shaming

73

you for your body, but it might be that your habits and lifestyle were influenced through your family, friends, and community. Sometimes we can identify where a particular message started to affect our mind.

I invite you to walk into your life with me and own your story and your body-image insecurity, as it is attached to your expectations and a prerequisite to self-worth and self-love. Your sense of worth lives inside your story. I am sure you have stories that don't fit with who you think you supposed to be, but not owning them gives shame an extraordinary power. The less you understand shame and how it affects your feelings, thoughts, and behaviors, the more power it exerts over your life. But when you speak about shame, you cut it of at its knees. You can't develop shame resistance, but you can develop shame resilience by walking into your stories and owning them. No wonder so many of us try diet after diet to get the body that is like a cultural requirement to feel good about ourselves. And it's no surprise that we feel shame about our bodies and that emotional eating can turn into an opportunity for shaming as well.

Most of the time, the reason we go on diets is to get control over our bodies. This is what we think consciously. With the dieting mind-set, you call days good or bad based on how you eat. That is, you can feel good and proud of yourself on any given day you eat well, based on your diet, and you feel bad and are hard on yourself when you eat something you shouldn't. On a bad day, you feel guilty or ashamed of yourself, and you put your self-worth on the line by saying something like, "I am bad because I ate this," or, "I am not good enough because I can't keep my diet."

A diet mentality is actually an area of shame on our body and eventually on our moral character.

Limiting beliefs can drive you to thinking that if you eat healthy today, you've earned the right to feel good about yourself; if you are able to do it right, you are valuable and worthy. But if you can't live up to these expectorations, it means that there is something wrong with you, and you must not be good. It is a total opportunity for judgment. This is how chronic dieters spend most of their time and energy every day, year round.

This is not a happy life to live. The diet mind-set teaches you to blame yourself for falling off your diets and teaches you to feel bad about yourself when you eat food that you are not supposed to consume. This is how we develop food shame and feel guilty around eating. The former is a real issue among women and girls that we need to be aware of. Every time you feel ashamed around eating, the shame will keep you feeling like you are flawed and insufficient.

Emotional weight can be seen as extra weight for protection, and you can now look at it as positive attention to help you let go of the guilt and shame.

The shameful feeling of not being able to stay on track with diets, not being able to keep from eating emotionally, or not preventing body-image insecurity is wrapped up with shameful feelings of inadequacy. Shame kills love, and judging yourself is not a practice of self-love.

I invite you to drop any shame you have around food, dieting, or emotional eating. Doing the diet-binge cycle can trigger you to feel ashamed if you are unable to control what you eat, and emotional eating can became a shaming minefield too. We think, "I am good if I don't eat emotionally," and, "I am bad" if I eat emotionally."

It might be difficult to accept this, but all the feelings of guilt, frustration, and shame around food are actually like messengers to tell you that something is out of alignment. You need to do something to feel centered and grounded again. I mentioned this in previous sections, but it's important enough to repeat it here.

I think it is crucial to acknowledge that shame can keep you in a box, and the only thing you feel you can do at that point is fight for your worthiness. Shame is a feeling of not being good enough, and that's one of the driving forces behind dieting, emotional eating, and body shame. You may eat the same food at a meal with a friend of yours, and while she can experience the food in its essence, you might be eating guilt and shame along with it. This is not a happy way to live.

How to Let Go of Shame

Shame and Its Role in Human Behavior

Brené Brown (Ph.D., L.M.S.W, is a writer, vulnerability and shame research professor) gives the following description: "Shame is the intensely painful feeling or experience of believing we are flawed and therefore unworthy of acceptance and belonging. Woman often experience shame when they are entangled in a web of layered, conflicting, and competing social-community expectations. Shame creates feelings of fear, blame, and disconnection."

For most of us, just thinking about becoming vulnerable and sitting with our feelings can bring up a visceral reaction. The antivulnerable upbringing can trigger a feeling of being ashamed if we want to show up with real emotions. One way practicing self-love is to get vulnerable. The answer lies within you.

Shame is rarely talked about, but understanding it is an important stepping-stone for someone who has weight struggles, a diet mentality, and body-image insecurity.

There are two different kinds of shame, and before I get into the applied shame that can suck the life out of you, let me share a bit about healthy shame.

Healthy Shame

Shame is one of the most important behavioral guides. It will save your life if you are about to do something idiotic. Shame is a key emotion in your social life and your inner life. It helps you to set boundaries and prevents you from breaking the boundaries of other people.

When shame is healthy, it helps you to turn away from thievery, even when no one is looking. It keeps you polite and will lead you to stop during temptation to do something that could shame you or shame others.

For example, in the moment that you are about to say or do something that would hurt somebody, shame can come up like a fire, turn your face red, and make you lose the capacity for speech.

Healthy shame is a gift in the form of supporting integrity, self-respect, and behavioral change.

Applied Shame

Getting vulnerable about how we feel and express our emotions is a huge act of courage in US society. Vulnerability means engaging in your life from a place of worthiness, where you let the world know about your needs and struggles regardless of what the outcome is. And that scares us like nothing else. It means you will get exposed. And the potential outcome of showing up in your life is that you might end up in a storm of applied shame from the outside world, including the environment you live in and the media at large.

We can't really get away from applied shame. It is how we raise children and how we train each other. But as we grow, we can find ways to oppose these external moral structures that try to impose shame.

Peeling Back the Layers of Applied Shame

We live in a society where different marketing strategies trigger us, emphasizing our flaws to make us choose to buy more products. When we do make those purchases, we feel good about ourselves and less flawed. Emotions like shame and guilt are often used in these contexts.

More specifically, social shaming or guilt tripping are often used as emotional marketing tools. The fear of being criticized, judged, and ridiculed by others has led to billions of dollars of products being sold.

The concept of social embarrassment isn't just a mix of mortification, indignity, and distress; it also consists of strategy and emotional marketing using shame and guilt.

For example, toothpaste ads suggest that with a fresh mouth you might attract a mate; by coloring your gray hair or having plastic surgery, you can look younger. There are skin-lightening products in the Philippines; the central message of the ads us that people who have lighter skin are more attractive and achieve greater success. It is a sign of wealth. Skin-whitening creams are sold in greater amounts than Coca-Cola in India. There used to be a time when body odor was not considered obnoxious or improper, so advertisers figured out a way to associate these odors with shame and then used this shame to sell a panacea.

Overall, the social shaming has become the selling strategy to make the most money of all time. Weight stigmas, body shame, and dieting are all interconnected terms in social embarrassment, but they are also a money-making factory.

Prior to the industrial revolution, before luxury goods and expensive items, most people lived rural existence on farms, grew their own food, and made their own clothes. Social positioning wasn't necessary. But as advancements emerged into our daily lives, people began judging and drawing conclusions about each other by what someone paid for and on personal appearance. As self-awareness grew in these areas, advertisers quickly took the opportunity to create marketing strategies; as a result, social positioning worked its way into advertising.

In present times, self-consciousness and the shame of not being good enough in appearance is in full swing. One example of applied shame is when women (or men) are told that their personal beauty is something that makes them better, stronger, or more worthwhile.

From breath, teeth whiteness, hair, and nails to lips or skin, you can hardly find an aspect of your appearance that can't be improved. One of the biggest target markets is young people, as they are the future market. Another big market has also been created, which is shaming people growing old. Endless marketing tools are directed to the older population to sell the idea that visibly growing old is not something to be celebrated. One of the biggest trends all over the world is cosmetic surgery. Although the industry emphasizes beauty and happiness, the underlying message is that if you don't follow the image offered in advertisements, you might get cast out by your peers. What is this if not shaming? And as the survival instinct of our subconscious mind wants to fit in, marketing creates not only shame but also fear.

Shame is used so often in marketing because applied shame creates anxiety in people, and everybody wants a solution to avoid being ashamed and feeling small. Wanting to avoid shame therefore fuels a need to not only create and sell but also to buy products that offer solutions for problems. And since less-than-perfect customers are the targets, marketing experts can create artificial needs by evoking guilt and shame in every human being. Products are the solution for these problems. Marketers created a shame-based culture because satisfied customers are not as profitable as discontented ones.

Shame is also used by people who feel they need to diet harder or work out more, but in general, shame is a negative motivator. It might motivate you to use willpower to diet and exercise, but eventually it doesn't feel good, and we give up. Self-loathing doesn't help us create long-term change, and it certainly doesn't keep us happy.

Letting go of shame and gaining self-acceptance are processes that go hand in hand. Although social expectations are not going to change anytime soon, if you are more aware of the emotional marketing you encounter on a daily basis, it is harder for feelings of inadequacy and pain to take over your mind and make you feel miserable. Don't let anyone define you. In fact, recent studies have shown that self-compassion is a much better motivator than shame for long-term changes. It soothes you when you need soothing, but you can keep yourself accountable.

When we are trapped in malfunctioning, repetitive, and unresolved shame, we are almost always responding to other people's ideas of what's right and wrong. This will cause us to eat, buy, and do the wrong things. Underneath our emotional eating patterns, the feeling of shame is undeniable.

Shame Gremlins

As Brené Brown calls it the "shame gremlin", which is a metaphor for the shame videos, also known mind chatter for the critical voice, the thoughts and conversations you have inside yourself. We all have this internal voice. Shame gremlins silence us. When we feel shame, we are taken back to a place of smallness where we lose a sense of context. We can't see anything else. When we are in shame, we don't accurately think about our strengths and limitations. We just feel alone, exposed, and deeply flawed. It is a human experience that is becoming increasingly pervasive, and it is a destructive part of our culture.

Shame sucks every ounces of light out of you until you are left feeling hopeless—feeling that nothing is good in your life. Some people have a visceral reaction to the word "shame" itself.

Shame drives you to feel two things:

- You'll never be good enough.
- Who do you think you are?

When it comes to applied shame, we all have it. It is a common human experience. People who don't feel it have no capacity for empathy or connection. However, we don't talk about shame. Nobody wants to. The less you talk about it, the more you feel it. We live in a culture of scarcity, and it is prone to making people experience shame. We have a tendency to feel ashamed not only if we don't have the perfect house, car, or body but also we use shame to dictate behavior in schools, family environments, and in society at large. In conversations, we use personal attacks and tear downs as a form of shaming. This is how we make ourselves heard. It is like we each have a motto on our forehead saying, "I am never … enough." You fill in the blank. For example, we are never thin enough, smart enough, beautiful enough, good enough, powerful enough, certain enough, perfect enough, extraordinary enough, or relevant enough. We live in a culture of scarcity. We have shame-based fears that if we don't acquire an extraordinary set of skills, our lives are worth nothing. We are hyper aware of our lack.

As impossible as it is to avoid applied shame, with the right tools you can help yourself recover from it. This recovery can save you from compulsive eating, body-image insecurity, and the constant struggle to be on a diet.

Think about how you feel physically when you are in shame. Usually people describe shame with the following symptoms: face flushes (turns red); palms, armpits, or bellybutton tingles; time slows down; stomach tightens; a choking sensation; nausea; can't breathe; feeling small; stomach drops; and inability to hold a gaze. Interestingly enough, these are actually trauma symptoms. We experience shame as trauma. Women who feel unworthy of love and belonging because of their inability to lose weight or manage their weight feel ashamed, and the threat of being unlovable is crazy-making. If you look at yourself in the mirror while you put on your pants and think you are not okay and instead feel ashamed for not having the body you are supposed to have, ask yourself the following question: Does your shame come from you, or does it come from your family, the media, or some other source?

If you want to get away from the suffering effects of self-doubt or self-abuse for not reaching those unattainable expectations, or if you are a silent victim of media attacks and teardowns, I invite you to use the following method of shame awareness and resilience when you are prone to feeling shame.

Practice Shame Resilience by Using This Three-Step Model

Applied shame resilience is a tool that can be used on a daily basis. You get so much relief, not because you changed your outside experience but because the hustle for worthiness is kind of pointless. You understand the world around you, and that gives you peace of mind.

1: Recognize Shame, Own It, and Share Your Story

There is a power in owning your story and reaching out. Shame is a very individualized and contextualized experience. Our families of origin—what we hear growing up—have a huge influence on our shame gremlins; our environmental, social, and cultural expectations also have a huge impact on our life.

When you run into applied shame, you have two choices: You walk into the stories of your life and own them because your worth lives inside your bigger story, or you stand outside your stories and hustle for your worth.

Remember, cultivating self-worth has to do with how you treat yourself. It has nothing to do with your strength and limitations. You are imperfectly perfect just the way you are.

We all have stories that we don't think fit into the person we think we are supposed to be, but not owning your stories gives shame extraordinary power. Therefore, the key to developing shame resilience is to walk into your stories and to own them.

When you acknowledge your story and share it with people who earned the right to hear it, shame dissipates.

As Brené Brown says, shame thrives in situations of secrecy, silence, and judgment, but the minute you share your story, the shame dies. When it meets empathy, shame disappears. By sharing your story, you also cultivate courage and strength. You simply stand up taller by walking your truth.

If you can say out loud, "This is who I am. I have all of these things that I am still working on, but I am okay. I respect and accept myself, even though there will be people who don't like or accept my story," you will stop hustling for your worthiness. Once you can shine the light on the darkness, it goes away.

You can have multiple shame triggers that start from your relationship with food, your body, and everything underneath. There is no problem too small in comparative suffering. Your problem is as important as anyone else's.

2: Be Aware of Your Thoughts and Feelings— Don't Overidentify with Them

It is important to take a balanced approach to negative emotions so that your feelings are neither suppressed nor exaggerated. Be aware of what's going on in your mind. Because you are a human, you will always have feelings, but that doesn't mean they are always right. Dr. Kristin Neff is a researcher and professor at the University of Texas at Austin. She runs the Self-Compassion Research Lab, where she studies how to develop and practice this skill to have a better approach to supporting ourselves and not beating ourselves up.

She uses mindfulness as a practice of self-compassion, which can be great when you are feeling shame. Mindfulness requires that you don't overidentify with thoughts and feelings to prevent being caught up and swept away by negativity. There is no way to live a happy life when you believe in your painful thoughts. That is, we are often unable to think clearly when we get stuck in our feelings. We make our emotions into facts, and our emotional state becomes reality. However, keep in mind that you are not your thoughts or emotions. You have them, but they don't define who you are. Observe them, but don't overidentify with them. Remember, you might have a problem, but you are not the problem itself.

3: Practice Critical Awareness Against Applied Shame

Critical awareness will evaluate expectations, including gender-specific expectations, you pick up from society and media. When you are in shame or you feel unworthy about your body or food, you are almost always responding to someone else's opinion about a certain issue. Appearance and body image is still the primary shame trigger for women, to this day. Society says we should do it all, do it perfectly, and look smoking hot while doing it.

As Brené Brown, shame researcher, points out, shame makes us feel small and unworthy. It can only thrive in silence and secrecy. Because of this, you have to acknowledge and share your feelings and story. It is healing. If you take a petri dish and put secrecy, silence, judgment, and empathy in it, you create a hostile environment for shame. Shame can't grow or thrive in the environment of empathy.

You can either own your story or keep hustling for worthiness. When you do the former, you get to choose the end. It's like you become a movie director. It can be difficult at first to rewrite a story because what you have gone through is painful, but if you do it, you can change the storyline. You can think of it like, "I am imperfect but totally loveable, and this is how the story ends." Can you feel the power of this approach?

How Do You Know When You Lose Applied Shame?

As I said earlier, I believe the most important thing is the need to drop shame around dieting, emotional eating, and body shame. Then you will be able to look behind these things and see why they are truly happening. You know you are good at dropping shame when the following could describe you:

- You don't comment on your moral character as a person no matter how your days turn out in the context of healthy eating or dieting
- You don't put your self-worth on the line regardless of how you feel about your body
- Eating emotionally and the reason for it don't create a shame spiral in you
- You don't self-identify or place your self-worth on what other people think about your body and how loveable you are based on that

I am not saying that you shouldn't stay responsible for your goals in nutrition. However, if you want to keep yourself accountable, judge the action, not yourself as a person. If you do eat emotionally or get off your diet on a given day, you can learn from it, but don't attack your self-worth or shame yourself, no matter how the day has gone.

Whether you struggle with dieting, emotional eating, or body shame, don't let the outside noise make you feel less worthy. Don't let anyone tell you that you are not worthy because you don't own certain things or don't have special traits. Recognize what's happening to you, and own the awareness you now have. If you pass a billboard that says you can only be as good as your flawless skin, skinny body, and so forth, catch your mean thoughts and bad feelings. You know that applied shame is present in modern society. However, shaming yourself or beating yourself up will not lead anywhere helpful. It only adds to your pain. The ideal form of beauty is different at different times. I am sure you can find a time in the past where your body type would be considered the ideal.

Therefore, whenever you can, catch shame regarding how you feel about your body. It is not always easy, even if you are aware how ridiculous the expectations are about how you are supposed to look. It can hurt even though you recognize and use shame resilience. But it can also feel like someone removed a hundred pounds from your shoulders when you realize how unfair the expectations are. Catch yourself when you apply all-or-nothing thinking because it means you still have a diet mentality regarding food consumption. Just because you eat something you are not supposed to, it doesn't make you a bad person. We humans are drawn to do things that feel good. There is a reason you do what you do: You only want to ease up on yourself. Drop shame so that we can start looking under the hood to see the root causes of your actions in the form of food shame and body shame.

Self-Care Skill Two: Check in with Your Mind Chatter

The Power of Beliefs
What you believe is what helps you achieve the greatness you are aiming for.

Socialization patterns and fundamental feelings of wanting to belong drive your belief system. Even when you grow up and move away from your family environment, you might feel a sense of disconnection in your decisions and in how you live your life based on the beliefs your family gave you. Fundamental feelings of belonging can show up in the form of fear of doing anything that challenges the beliefs system you are used to—anything that challenges the status quo.

Starting the next diet or eating compulsively always reveals the belief you have. These actions tell others (and yourself) about your core beliefs. When you choose to eat compulsively, triggered by what you believe is true, you are also communicating, "I have no other choice but to eat."

As you grow older, you are becoming more aware of how you feel and what you need based on your emotions. Aside from this, you also develop a voice of authority as part of your developmental process. In the chapter "Losing Self-Worth from Family of Origin," I lay down the foundation of your core beliefs regarding your self-worth.

The inner voice I call "mind chatter" can be nurturing and accepting, and it can also be critical or judgmental. It can feel like an enemy lives inside of you with a shaming voice, not a soothing one.

You develop and pick up this inside voice, your "mind chatter," from your environment. It can be influenced by things such as how people have treated you, how you see people treating themselves, the expectations you get from life and society, and how you are treated based on how you perform. This process is called "introjection," and it is about the expectations, projections, of others—that is, the way they communicate nonverbally and verbally or covertly and overtly. As you grow up, you naturally look to your environments to define you. Good emotional and mental health is based on getting your needs met in a certain period of your life. Anyone with compulsive behavior around dieting or emotional eating most likely doesn't know how to meet those needs without distraction.

The moment you can step away from your inner critic and approach uncomfortable feelings with gentleness, self-compassion, and kindness, you point your attention toward the underlying issues. The "inner critique," or mind chatter, is only the mirror of your environment— family, friends, or teachers. But it defines you as an authority. The inner critic only tries to keep you away from abandonment and able to maintain your relationship with those whom you are dependent on.

The system almost of us grew up with was mostly based on one thought: When you were good, you got love, but when you misbehaved, your caregivers withdrew love to get what they wanted. Obviously, it shouldn't be like this, but most parents are this way. Now, let's start focusing on how to go forward.

If people around you were supportive and understanding as you grew up, there is a higher chance you developed a voice of inner nurturing. If you were thought to have a sense of self-worth regardless of how you performed, there is a much higher change that you will have a nurturing relationship with yourself later in life. In contrast, if your environment was critical, unkind, or judgmental, and your community withdrew love based on how you performed—you thought it was your fault for not being lovable—most likely you developed an inner critic, a voice that beats you up, making you feel lonely and inadequate.

Your inner world reflects how you feel about yourself regardless of how the outside world perceives you. When you have a positive sense of self-worth, the emphasis is on how you treat yourself no matter what your strength and limitations are. Your mind chatter can help you restore your emotional balance if needed as an inner nurturer.

The biggest obstacle to any transformation can be what you believe to be the truth about yourself. According to cognitive therapy and developmental psychologists, we humans develop distorted thought patterns and self-defeating thoughts as we develop a fully operative voice inside of us. This happens by the time we are four years old. By the time we grow up, we stop being afraid of our caregivers and start paying attention the inner critic.

This voice always shows up when you want to move away from the status quo. It is especially loud if you were not raised with self-nurturing skills. When you want to challenge what your parents did, what you saw growing up, and the daily habits you acquired during your early years, the inner critic will always try to make you question the step you are about to take.

Why You Always Gain Weight Back

Picture this: You lose weight for the hundredth time, and now you have the body of your dreams. This is what you always wanted and envisioned, and now it is finally yours.

But when you look at yourself in the mirror, you realize that what you once considered perfect regarding your body shape is now reality, as you expanded your vision into your current state. Once we reach our goals, we immediately look to the next one for satisfaction. So, what you will see in the mirror is that you can always find a little part of you that says, "I should get a bit leaner here or lose a bit more there." Or the voice might say, "Wow, I actually look pretty good now. I hope can keep it up and not indulge in too much food. Since you think your self-worth is based on your thinness, when you reach your ideal weight, you realize that the only thing you can think about is how to stay thin. You can't seem to stop worrying.

It is shocking to see that a thin person can have the same victim mentality and experience with weight discrimination from a different point of view as when he or she was heavier. Once you are thin, shame triggers and the "syndrome of hating yourself can come to the surface by being afraid of gaining weight because we have the cultural idea that fat is bad and thin is good.

Remember how once you learned to swim, you wanted to learn how to swim faster? Similarly, as soon as you have the perfect body and should finally be happy, you start focusing on maintaining your weight to stay happy. Doesn't this sound crazy?

Our whole life is an ever-changing reality, and the only thing you actually have is the present moment and how you treat yourself in that moment. You can't be in the future or the past. If you chase tomorrow for your happiness, you miss out on today. You miss the opportunity to be happy right now. We think we don't like ourselves because we don't believe our body is good enough, and even though we spent way too much energy thinking about it and working on it, what happens a lot of the time is that you lose weight and still have insecurities and thoughts of not being good enough. This leads you to keep heading toward the diet-binge cycle or emotional eating pattern.

If you are a chronic dieter or compulsive eater and have spent the last five years, twenty years, or more losing and gaining weight, you might realize by now that something is going on. You may even suspect, accurately, that this has nothing to do with weight and everything to do with your life.

Even if you successfully lose weight by using your willpower to live by a diet plan and exercise regime for the fiftieth time, the thoughts, beliefs, and emotions forming the reasons you gained weight in the first place will still be there. The situations that triggered you to turn to food originally will still be there. In other words, as mentioned previously, the things that drove you to eat will show up on the surface when you are done with the diet plan that helped you lose weight. The feelings of unworthiness, inadequacy, loneliness, or being misunderstood will still be there, as will the desire to again wipe out these emotions with food or something else.

Dieting, soothing, or numbing with food has more to do with the fact that you are not happy with yourself as a person rather than the fact that you are not happy with your body. That is, the food, exercise, and body issues that make you unhappy with your body exist because you are actually unhappy with yourself. Therefore, your job in your weight, food, and body image struggle is to challenge old beliefs. This will lead to eye-opening experiences regarding how you think about yourself and your environment.

Feeling Fat Is Not a Feeling That You Experience as a Physical Sensation

What does it mean when you feel fat? I wonder how many times you have been in a situation when you are not even thinking about your weight or shape, and then something happens, and then sudden thoughts come up, such as, "I am fat," "I'm ugly," "I hate my body," and so on. The sudden experience of feeling fat is a product of your mind that is triggered by not being able to meet certain expectations; you find yourself in self-hate, self-doubt, and insecurity. Your self-worth is on the line, and uncertainty is the driving force making you feel that way. Please try to understand intellectually that you didn't gain weight in the last five seconds. It's not a physical sensation of weight gain. The feeling might not go away, but now you understand it intellectually, which can be helpful.

Whenever you have the thought of feeling fat, remember that it goes back to issues having to do with the quest for worth going on underneath. And this way of thinking is not your fault. Your struggle to accept your body and the perceived need for constant dieting because you think you are not good enough is the product of cultural conditioning and a product of your default core beliefs.

You are culturally conditioned to believe your worth has to do with your body size, and this is not truly who you are. In other words, the mental connection between feeling out of alignment with yourself and taking it out on your body is the product of living in modern society.

Next time you experience feeling fat, ask yourself the following questions:

- If I wasn't thinking about my weight and how fat I am, what would I be thinking about? What in my life makes me feel stress right now?
- What's taking up my mind at this moment? Where do I feel insecure, nervous, or inadequate?
- What's really bothering me right now?

When you carry yourself with pride and respect, the way you speak about yourself and treat yourself changes. It shows not only that you have a strong sense of self-worth but also the extent you are capable of actually loving yourself as you love others.

Until you recognize your own value, it is hard to find inner peace. We all have useless beliefs that tell us we are bad, we are not good enough, or we are unlovable. You are not alone in experiencing these thoughts. Understanding what's going on underneath feeling fat—the shame, fear, nervousness, guilt, anxiety, and so on—is half the battle. You don't need to buy a new wardrobe, thinking you are fat, every time negative emotions toward yourself and your body arise. All the expectations that culture puts on you have created this thought in your mind.

Change Your Relationship with Food: Take Care of Your Emotional Wounds

We go through life, experiencing different types of pain in our life. Physical injuries are treated and healed on a daily basis. When you break your leg or scrape your elbow against something, you learn about the ways to treat these physical injuries. What about common emotional injuries? Why can't we just get some wisdom about our experiences and move on with self-worth intact? Unfortunately, emotional health is often a second citizen compared to physical health. We have the idea that the way we should handle feelings is by not having them—or pretending not to have them.

However, as previous sections of this book have already alluded to, reasons for yo-yo dieting, body image issues, and emotional eating are all about understanding your true self—your thoughts and beliefs.

Every day, psychological injuries happen to all of us. We get wounded, and we don't take care of our emotional health. We generally only know what we are taught, and most of us learn to be tough and self-critical instead of attending to or showing your hurt feelings. This is also how we wired: We want to get away from our feelings. We don't want to feel uncomfortable.

In his book *Emotional First Aid*, Guy Winch discusses how everyday psychological injuries don't get treated, as we hold on to them. Emotional cuts such as rejection, failure, loneliness, damaged self-esteem, loss and traumas, and ruminating are all examples of the frequent issues we have to deal with. Chances are that if you are an emotional eater, you might be spinning the emotional hamster wheel instead of solving your problem.

Emotional wounds can send you back in time and make you experience a trauma again that happened in the past. You need to train your brain by changing your beliefs and recognizing that the memories are not your present reality; they don't present danger anymore. As you clear yourself from these emotional burdens by becoming aware and releasing the energy that those words affected you with, painful memories will lose their power over you.

One time I was checking out pictures of my friends on Facebook. And then suddenly I wanted to eat chocolate immediately and a lot of it. I knew I was out of emotional balance. I immediately stood up and headed for the kitchen; after eating a couple of bites of chocolate, I had a sense of relief. I didn't go into a full binge; instead, I questioned what was happening and dug deep. I realized that jealousy and judgment made me want to binge. My friends had something I didn't have. It seemed like they were all having fun, and I wasn't. I attached the emotional significance to those pictures that I didn't have the courage to enjoy life because I had so much going on; I felt that fun and play couldn't be part of my life if I wanted reach my goals. I knew that the only way I could ease my emotional pain around the photographs was to have the courage to understand what made me react the way I did.

Emotional pain arises from holding onto beliefs that can sabotage our goals in life, including weight-loss goals. A lot of times, judgments we form about others are reflections of our beliefs about ourselves and serve as a straitjacket to self-sabotaging behaviors like compulsive eating. These judgments can therefore create a block to our own success.

I was raised on the model that hard work pays off, but the idea that I could have fun at the same time was not part of that model. So I judged people who were having fun, thinking they were doing something wrong and would get nowhere in life. At the same time, my body and my heart yearned for play.

I eventually learned that when we judge people, it is like teaching your subconscious mind that it's not safe for you to have what those people have, because you may be judged in the same way you are judging them.

In my situation, I realized that while looking at those pictures on Facebook and judging my friends, I was creating a belief system for myself that it was not safe to work hard and have some fun in my life at the same time. And by believing this idea, I was constantly finding ways in my life to prove my value through struggling with long hours of work. I knew I had to change this belief system and understand that it was okay to have fun, even if I am an adult; by this point, I didn't feel jealous of my friends anymore. And adding more fun into my life didn't push me to binge on chocolate. In fact, it did quite the opposite.

Catch Self-Defeating Thoughts

You were not born feeling negative about yourself. Growing up, we all adopt and accept negative beliefs about ourselves our immediate environment provides, including our caregivers, our school environment, and the media. This is the time to understand that the beliefs you adopted are just someone else's opinions. As adults we have a tendency to settle into our beliefs and associate belief systems with who we are. Your work now is to challenge the beliefs you have adopted and no longer serve you. Critical thinking is important. However, most of us were not taught to evaluate our negative beliefs, regardless how they make us feel. Be like a child again, and don't be afraid to ask why regarding old beliefs. You can replace them with new beliefs that serve you and feel good.

The moment you catch and ponder self-defeating thoughts, you are creating new habits. You need to have the attitude of being aware that you are breaking the habit of dealing with your inner critic and not letting it ruin your life. If you let it run the show in your mind, you end up eventually focusing on whatever your inner critique tells you. If you want to make major changes in your life, you must not only take care of the underlying causes of your dieting patterns or emotional eating but also want to understand the thoughts and beliefs that lead you to suffer from body image insecurities or unwelcome feelings.

Be gentle and understanding with yourself. Don't beat yourself up; that's not a good motivator. Understand that if you don't want to suffer, you have to change what's not working for you. And spending years if not decades hating your body and working to get a new one or pushing down emotions but still feeling miserable is most likely a definite sign that something is not working for you. Instead of hating yourself, focus on creating a life you want to lead. Focus on how you want to feel.

Similar to the fact that hating people doesn't get them to love you, you can only drop your emotional weight for good by loving yourself. You have to try to understand who you are without all the beliefs that lead you to chronic dieting, body shame, or compulsive eating.

To engage in this process, ask yourself the following questions:

- Where and when did I learn that I'm not good enough, pretty enough, smart enough, or beautiful enough?
- What events, people, and messages do I use to support my negative feelings about myself?

I meet women who want to lose weight very badly but are also afraid of the outcome. What will people think about them? Will they get more attention that makes them uncomfortable? Will people think they are shallow because of their pretty looks? The memories and emotional charges of past experiences can get in the way of transforming your body and your life. Clearing emotional residue from painful memories is the only path to successful and permanent body change.

Ask yourself the following questions regarding your weight:

- What's the benefit to you for holding on to weight?
- What's the downside of losing weight?
- What happened the last time you lost weight?

It is important to be aware of what you believe about yourself because it defines where you are in life. You must understand not just what you think consciously but also subconsciously. As discussed previously, many of your thoughts and beliefs come from the environment you live in and are there without your conscious awareness. Which program runs in your mind on a daily basis: the one that people expect you to have, or the one you think you deserve and want to have? The one that believes your happiness doesn't have to come in the form of expectations provided by the media, society, friends, or family? If do not examine what subconsciously runs on the video of your mind, telling you that you are not worthy enough, good enough, tall enough, or small enough, you will end up acting out of that belief system and not what is the truest version of yourself.

I left home when I was eighteen years old without having any specific faith. I didn't even know what the word meant. Religion and spiritualty were not things we discussed at home, and I didn't understand the concept of going to church, praying, or believing in anything that the eyes cannot see. However, I still left home with different tapes running in my mind. Some beliefs helped me on my way, but others didn't. For me, to let go of my body shame, I had to accept my body regardless of what society or people I knew thought of it. I stopped believing all the videos running in my mind because of the weight stigmas I got during my time as a professional dancer. I learned to love myself when I didn't feel like it. I learned to love myself when others didn't love me. And I learned to love myself when I felt no one could. When I was able let go my self-sabotaging mind chatter and make myself believe I deserved good things in my life no matter what others thought of me, somehow I attracted people into my life who supported this belief. I got rid of all the people in my life who judged my body and my appearance. I wish I had known then what I know now: People reflect their insecurities on others, so by judging me, these people were revealing their insecurities about their bodies. But because I deeply believed that I deserved good things in my life no matter what my body size was, I overcame a deeply seated conditioning.

You can take a journey of self-reflection to better understand your mental or emotional conditioning. The shift happens when you can choose a better way of life. All the nagging feelings you have about your worth regarding your body or anything that pushes you to relieve your emotions with food can be shifted or changed if you listen to your inner guidance.

You might not have learned how to nurture yourself when you were younger, but you can learn how to do it now. You can adapt your belief system so that you know you can have everything and be everything that you want in your life; if you can't get what you want, it's because there is something better for you. Only when you have a belief system and your worth is aligned with your inner value can you make those desires stick. If you are living in a space where you fear you are not good enough or worthy enough or can't have something, even affirmations and mantras will not work. They are only part of the package.

Your beliefs drive your behavior. Catherine Collautt, PhD, is a practicing philosopher, writer, metaphysician, and manifesting consultant. Her work centers on the subconscious mind. She says, "The subconscious mind, which works like an automatic pilot, is by far our greatest processing powerhouse. Scientists will tell you that the power of the subconscious mind is perhaps a million times greater than the conscious mind. This is not to say that your conscious mind does nothing, but I am pointing out how important it is to get the two aligned. You are meant to be the boss, managing the asset of your subconscious mind by giving it clear and good direction." Unfortunately, it doesn't matter how much you say you want to lose weight, stay thin, be brave, or have success; if you believe somewhere deep inside that managing your weight, getting off diets, or stop emotionally eating equals some kind of pain (loss of love, guilt, rejection, embarrassment, shame, or vulnerability) you will not let yourself do what it takes to succeed.

Let Go of Old Core Beliefs

First Step: Awareness—Identify Your Limiting Beliefs and Recognize Resistance

Most of the time, we don't want to get over our limiting beliefs because we are afraid of the metaphorical dark. We humans crave certainty, so we fear the unknown, and we fear being wrong. Social conditioning is so connected to limiting beliefs that you need to intentionally work with your resistance, not against it.

Your job is to catch the self-defeating thoughts you acquired via conditioning of modern times and examine them. James Allen, a British philosophical writer, once said, "The outer conditions of a person's life will always be found to reflect their inner beliefs. Once you master your beliefs you will master your life."

I have gone into great detail in this book to describe how the influence of family, culture, and media messages can twist your beliefs about what you are capable of reaching. Now it is your turn to be aware of these issues and to consider your self-defeating thoughts. Identify any limiting beliefs you have about yourself.

Don't assume that past events will predict future events. In reality, your current beliefs will predict the future. Your story is the end product of the choices you have made, based on the beliefs you have at any particular moment. Therefore, as soon as you change your beliefs, you are headed toward a change in your life story.

To help yourself recognize and let go of limiting beliefs, ask yourself the following questions:

What limiting belief am I holding on to?
I am not good enough to …
I am not worthy enough to …
I am only here to …

When you identify your internal response to completing the latter three sentences, listen to the wisdom in the resistance. Be humble, and don't judge it. Trust your subconsciousness long enough to learn from it.

The story you tell yourself about why you can't lose weight or stay thin will unfold in front of you if you do the work you need to do. Your job is to question your current belief system about your struggle, especially if it is telling you something that keeps you from reaching your goals. Whether the belief you're holding on to is that you can only lose weight if you push yourself or that weight loss is only for people who are genetically blessed, it is keeping you in a victim mode. It is time for you to search for an approach that will get you where you want to be.

Second Step: Release Your Limiting Beliefs

So, how do you change beliefs? Challenge their validity and then release them.

To start this process, ask yourself the following questions:

What is the fear (or what are the fears) I have, exactly?
What is it exactly that my subconscious mind is looking out for?
What expectations am I comparing myself to?
Am I comparing myself to others?
Where am I attacking myself?

The purpose of these questions is to interview your subconscious mind with genuine curiosity and self-compassion. You want it to make its case. It is not enough to identify that you don't feel good enough for such and such a reason; you need to know specifics about why you think the way you do.

You want to stay willing, witnessing the thoughts. Look for details and applaud whatever you find without judging it. Be willing to change and release the fear of whatever limiting belief you are holding on to.

When I was living my life in constant fear of being not good enough, it was partly because of my body image insecurity. I was the victim of internalized weight stigma and weight discrimination. Wanting to stay lean was part of my job because I was a professional dancer. Although I stopped dancing when I was twenty-one and started working behind the camera in television, the constant struggle to be thin still consumed my thoughts. All of the girls around me wanted to get skinnier and were on diets all the time. Looking back on those days, I realize that I did what looked normal because everybody was doing it. I totally fell for the notion that staying lean could get me the guy and the happiness I wanted for myself. And the sad thing is that I attracted guys whose priority was to only date thin girls, so my staying skinny was a big deal for them. One time I was down to eighty pounds, and I got an appreciative look from an ex-boyfriend as he said that I looked my best. And I was proud and happy about the comment until I met one of my friends on the street, and her shocking look told me something was wrong. She said that I looked like an anorexic, and she was worried about me.

It is mind-blowing for me to look back and see that I had a life wherein I was a victim of weight discrimination and the beliefs that create it. I was only one of the many women who felt that unless we had the perfect body, we couldn't have a great career, a nice boyfriend, or an awesome life. Accepting discrimination against the so-called normal body shape and weight is an unspoken social requirement. We are so worried about not fitting in that we don't even realize how much we perpetuate the cultural bias wherein extra weight means you are lazy or stupid. When I started to question the validity of my beliefs, only then I was able to release them because I recognized that they didn't serve me at all. I set myself free from the life sentence I had previously given myself.

You can always find the good in your beliefs and change your perception. Life is like a mirror. People who hurt you are like teachers. They show up in your life to help you learn something, and as soon as you pass through their presence and change your perception, your belief system will eventually change too. This allows you to be in the same situation but look, think, and feel about it from a very different point of view. This can lead to happiness, even if the circumstances haven't changed.

At the time, I unconsciously looked for evidence to support my old belief that I was only good enough to date if I had a thin body. I downplayed positive feedback and resonated with negative feedbacks— not because anyone who said I was fat was right, but because I believed what they said. I gave my power away to those who criticized me.

The most mind-blowing thing about situations when we accept weight discrimination or weight stigmas from others is that most likely they also have unresolved issues or insecurities with their bodies. They are only projecting those on to us. And we take it personally and let it define us. Of course, this couldn't be further from the truth. But again, our core beliefs make us believe that feedback. If even a tiny part of us thinks these people are not right but you still get criticism about your body, you will believe their statements are valid but refuse to be treated disrespectfully.

Byron Katie said, "Our parents, our children, our spouse, and our friends will continue to press every button we have, until we realize what it is that we don't want to know about ourselves, yet. They will point us to our freedom every time."

It's time to discover what events you are using from your life to proof that you are not good enough.

Self-Care Skill Three: Feel and Let Go of the Resistance

Emotions and Vulnerability

If you are an emotional eater, you put your feelings into food instead of feeling and dealing with them. This reaction to emotions not only supports your struggle with compulsive eating but also stops you from managing your weight. You need to understand and acknowledge that you use compulsive eating, in the form of binging, overeating, or chronic dieting as a shield against vulnerability so you don't have to show up with real emotions.

Interestingly enough, we typically work with nutrition and exercise to increase our energy, but we ignore the richest source of energy we possess: our emotions. We are intellectually brilliant, physically resourceful, and spiritually imaginative but emotionally underdeveloped. This is a shame, because emotions contain vitality that can be channeled toward self-knowledge, one of the keys to stopping emotional eating and weight struggles. Unfortunately, emotions are more often categorized, celebrated, vilified, repressed, manipulated, humiliated, adored, and ignored. Rarely, if ever, are they honored.

Emotional eating can cause health problems. Even though it feels good at the moment, it carries risk because it is about repressing healthy emotions. Expressing our feelings in an appropriate and timely manner is essential for mental and physical health. In contrast, holding emotions in leads to a buildup of negativity and discomfort inside of us, and it can often show itself in the form of stress, feeling tense, or being resentful of other people without fully realizing why.

Using food to anesthetize or cope with feelings also means that we tend to ignore problems that need attention. For example, if we eat when we are bored, lonely, or angry with someone, how does that help resolve the issue? When frequently eating to cope with our emotions and the beliefs behind them, we can develop a bad relationship with food. Specifically, reacting to emotions with food often leads to compulsive overeating, binge eating, chronic dieting, bulimia, and anorexia. Your body can suffer from a whole range of resulting medical complications. If you are relying on eating as your single coping mechanism for all the stressors in your life, it means you don't have an effective toolbox or to help you deal with different situations.

I am sure you can see by now that there is a connection between mood states and eating. As previously described, when emotions come up, instead of feeling and discharging them, you instead choose a coping mechanism, which is eating. You are significantly undernourished in your emotional guidance system because you don't have a menu of emotional management options to naturally express your emotions in the right time, at the right place. Your emotions drive you toward unhealthy behaviors, such as compulsive eating. Compulsive eating has multiple reasons, but lack of emotional flow is the bottom line.

Emotional imbalance triggers reactive eating, which in turn results in comforting with food, and this is not even the real issue. Compulsive eating and weight fluctuations are here to tell you something. I know it's hard to listen; the end of the road seems invisible and uncertain. But I am here, setting the pace for you, and I will get you there. I have been on your side for a long time, and although it took me some time to get past this behavior, it is possible. But I need you to be brave, to have the courage to truly feel and express your emotions. Searching for what lies behind these behaviors is quite a journey. It is a process wherein your conscious and subconscious mind will meet with your emotions.

As previously mentioned, chronic weight fluctuation, permanent weight-loss resistance, chronic dieting, and emotional eating are an external reflection of a deep internal problem. Discovering the real issue and learning how to release the need that causes the excess weight is now our goal.

Start by asking yourself what emotional weight you are carrying around.

Otherwise healthy women and girls who are on and off diets for at least a couple of years and whose weight fluctuates all the time deal with an issue that is about more than just nutrition. As discussed previously, there is a connection between mood, emotions, and eating patterns. There can be multiple reasons you eat compulsively. When you use your willpower and extreme focus for a period of time to work off your unwanted weight, you often ignore the reasons you gained it in the first place.

It is empowering to understanding who you are in your emotions, as they wrap around all your decisions, your dreams, your fears, and your desires. It is also the only solution to chronic weight fluctuation.

Compulsive eating is a powerful and unhealthy coping mechanism, even though it temporarily saves our sanity. Every time we try to only treat the symptom, the compulsive eating, we miss the point.

When you have light bulb moments and you are aware of what fuels your emotional eating, that's when the real work begins. Finding the root cause that drives your cravings often means you need to override your old beliefs and to make difficult choices for the better. If you can recognize what's missing in your life and work toward a more fulfilling future, you'll find it much easier to make the right choices when it comes to food. Eventually, it will become effortless.

Understanding Feelings

We humans all want to feel good about ourselves and find joy, happiness, and satisfaction. Our inborn need is to feel aligned with ourselves, centered, content, comfortable, and at peace. Our emotions are what connect us to ourselves, and so the level of connection can only be strong if our belief and feelings are aligned with who we really are.

Gary Zukav, graduate of Harvard University and author of *The Seat of the Soul*, says, "Without an awareness of our emotions, we cannot associate the effects of anger, sadness, grief and joy—within ourselves or others—with their causes. When we close the door to our feelings, we close the door to the vital currents that energize and activate our thoughts and actions. We cannot begin the process of understanding the effect of our emotions upon us, our environment, and other people, or the effects of the emotions of other people upon themselves, their environment, and us."

Feelings are like our canary in the coal mine. If you want to create a life that feels good to you, first you need to be able to experience your feelings. And you can't be selective about which emotions you feel. To know what true happiness is, you need to also learn what anger and pain is.

As discussed previously, compulsive eaters react to emotions with food and can't lose weight or manage it permanently because they don't understand their feelings. They don't really know how to express them or move past them without eating. So, when their emotional well-being is at risk, it puts them on a fast track to consume comfort foods.

To come back to emotional alignment without food, you need to connect to your own inner guidance. And this requires vulnerability—the willingness to feel what you sense and not push down your emotions. Although we can't choose to have feelings or not, because that comes with being a human, we can choose the ways we digest them. That is, we can choose to comfort ourselves another way and move past our feelings without eating.

What's interesting about trying to avoid emotional discomfort is that we are pretty much hardwired to ignore pain physically and psychologically. Pain, no matter what kind, signals that something is wrong, and it triggers the fight, flight, or freeze response in us. You feel pain, and you associate it with a problem and want to get away from it as much as possible. It's very useful as a protective factor, but that's the same reason so many people shut themselves off from their emotions.

What's fascinating about emotional imbalances is that they push you to connect with yourself and the world around you. It's like somebody or something is giving you signals from the inside that something is out of whack. They say, *Hey girl, what's up? What's driving you crazy, making you happy, sad, anxious, and so forth?*

Emotions are vilified as signs of weakness in our culture. Throughout the discussion in this book, you realize by now that one of the keys to overcoming weight struggles and compulsive eating is to understand your emotions and learn to flow with them instead of pushing them down with food.

What Is an Emotion?

Antonio Damasio, neuroscientist, says that emotions are "action requiring neurological programs." If you can look at emotions by the definition, you can turn toward them rather than running away. You can ask what action they require from you so that you can develop a brand new relationship with the emotion and access the skills, gifts, and abilities it brings you rather than treating it as something that happens to you. Since our body is made up of moving energetic particles, we are destined to feel emotions and feelings fully and then let them pass through us.

What's the Difference between Emotions and Feelings?

Emotions tend to be in your mind, when you understand that you experience sadness, happiness, anxiety, fear, hurt, shame, or anger.

Feelings, in contrast, are the physical sensation of all of your emotions. For example, when most people are happy, they feel it in their heart—their chest. When anxious, some people feel it in their whole body or in their shoulders and back. The location and intensity that each person experiences feelings is unique.

Emotions are a form of energy that needs to be expressed, as it has a particular vibration in the body. Everything in the universe has a vibration. Each rock and tree has its own vibration. Each type of cell and organ also has its own vibration. Awareness of these currents is the first step in learning how your experiences come into being and why. The only emotion you can heal is the one that you let yourself feel and express. Emotions are the physical vibration of what you hold onto. For example, if you are kind to someone or you feel happy, your level of vibration is higher than if you feel worried, disappointed, or sad. In other words, negative and positive emotions change the frequency of your vibration all the time. Different thoughts create different emotions, hence different vibrations in your body. If you can't or don't express your emotion, it is pushed down in your body and sits within you. If you are emotionally blocked, you might not even know what you feel, and you become kind of dull and negative.

By learning to use the language of emotions, we can identify how we feel and give ourselves a chance to express it. You need to have the willingness to truly experience what you feel. You give an emotion power by putting energy into suppressing it. Take a couple of deep breaths, feel the emotion in your body, acknowledge it, and then let it pass through you. To overcome ongoing weight struggles, it is essential to feel your feelings but not wallow in them or overidentify with them. It is okay to cry and laugh, even if you were taught that it is not okay. Feelings and emotions are like reset buttons for humans. They give us relief. We are a species that makes meaning, wired to seek understanding of our emotions, thoughts, and behaviors and those of others. Have you ever thought about how different emotions can bring you clarity and strength? They provide information, so when they come knocking on your door, don't run and hide, pretending no one is home. Let them come to you so that when they pass, you can get back to a more positive vibration.

Feeling your feelings instead of eating them requires engaging in your life. Listen to your inner guidance from your emotions and feelings about your needs, wants, and desires. Feel and share them instead of hiding and numbing them. When you run away from shame, embarrassment, fear, guilt, or humiliation, you are headed toward your artificial saving grace, which is binging and numbing.

We Are Emotional Beings, Longing for Connection and Belonging

Abraham Maslow, American psychologist, argued that the human needs for individual growth and happiness can't be met without first satisfying a more basic need, human connection. For us to achieve our full potential as human beings, love and affection are primary needs. Many other psychologists supported this theory. Heinz Kohut, psychoanalyst, who developed a model called "self-psychology," proposed that belongingness was one of the core needs of the self.

We are wired to love, to be loved, and to belong. When those needs are not met, we don't function as we were meant to. We break and fall apart. We numb ourselves. We ache. We hurt others. We get sick.

Interestingly enough, when I have my clients write a food journal to record their emotions right before and after a binge, they often write about their thoughts rather than their feelings or emotions.

One of the most difficult parts for most people who struggle with permanent weight-loss and emotional eating is the struggle to be willing to look behind the curtain and feel their emotions. Opening up and letting your feelings come to the surface can be intimidating.

Emotions and Vulnerability

When you disconnect from your emotions, it means you don't want to be vulnerable. You miss the opportunity to connect with how you feel and what you really need. When you push down your feelings, for example with food, your world can become meaningless, empty, and lonely.

If you do this, it's because you think about vulnerability as a negative emotion like fear, shame, grief, uncertainty, or risk, and you choose not to engage these emotions. This is how we protect ourselves from things we don't want to feel.

Based on our socialization process, a lot of us grew up with a belief that showing emotions was not what strong or cool people do. In our civilization, for some reason, we have an idea that not just showing feelings but feeling them is a weakness.

It is almost a universal belief that vulnerability is a dark emotion and the birthplace of all the feelings and emotions we don't want to feel—fear, uncertainty, shame, grief, and disappointment. It's like saying, "I don't want to be vulnerable because that means I am uncertain, afraid, weak, or exposed." We don't want to show up with real feelings and emotions, even with ourselves. So, we armor up against vulnerability and head to the bottom of an ice-cream carton.

The truth is that although vulnerability is the center of difficult emotions, it is also the birthplace of every positive emotion we need in our lives: love, joy, belonging, happiness, and empathy. Vulnerability is life itself. How can you live without it if you want to live your life fully? Honestly, if you don't practice vulnerability, you will binge and eat emotionally for the rest of your life.

But for now, let us look closer at how vulnerability can save your ass and your life. It saved mine, for sure. When we were young, many of us had to tough it out and not show emotions. That's what our caregivers modeled and passed on to us. Vulnerability can be defined as uncertainty, risk, and emotional exposure. Vulnerability is also about letting ourselves be seen. If you were lucky while growing up, your family environment was supportive enough to let you be vulnerable and express your emotions. But the world, especially media-driven expectations and the cultural environment, is very supportive of individualism. They tell you not to share your insecurities with others, because you might lose face. Instead, do it perfectly.

When I asked clients about how much attention they paid to their emotions and if they access and express them, I got answers like the following: "Showing emotions means becoming vulnerable, and it is more like looking weak, acting stupid, or leaning into joy can look uncool." They told me how difficult or embarrassing it would be for them to show emotions, so they preferred to push them down or avoid them. Whether they restricted food or overate, instead of taking care of their emotions, they used food to get control over the feelings. They used it to take the edge off their powerless thoughts and feelings and to fill up the inner emptiness.

It is important to understand that unless you are willing to work and understand the emotions that lead you to overeat, binge, or numb certain feelings, you can't and will not stop yo-yo dieting. As I mentioned before, going on and off diets can be the effect of restricting yourself from certain foods, but it's also because your emotions drive you to eat. It has nothing to do with your physical hunger, because the problem you are trying to solve—the ongoing dieting effect—is partly created by your emotions.

As the body detoxifies itself via various channels (sweating, breathing, going to the restroom, etc.), you also need to detoxify and work through your feelings.

Becoming vulnerable and expressing your emotions is a normal part of life. You were trained not to do it. However, you can never outgrow the need to feel and express your emotions. It is a basic human need. There are a couple of myths surrounding vulnerability that we can explore in more depth. The interesting thing about myths is that the truth is often the opposite of that which we assume to be real.

I believe that one of the most important elements of ending your weight issues is to be daring enough to became vulnerable and show up in regard to your emotions at the right time and place. Therefore, let's examine some myths about vulnerability and how this trait can actually help you to put together the puzzle of your life.

Myth 1: Only Weak People Are Vulnerable

Childhood and Adolescence

Most of us grew up struggling with feelings of shame, unworthiness, and fear of some sort. If you grew up in a nurturing environment, social or cultural expectations may have pushed you into feeling these same things. Overall, most of us experience some type of insecurity, and we get the impression from our environment that it is not safe to be vulnerable because that's not what smart, strong, cool people do, just like my clients related. So we build walls to feel safe. We shut down part of ourselves for this protection. We decide we are not going to put ourselves out there because it can be intimidating, and we might lose our positive self-image. We are not really open to risk.

Adult Life

But in our adult lives, we realize that the people we want to be as parents, friends, and professionals, we need to engage in our life and let ourselves be seen. The heartwrenching reality is realizing that we need to tear down those walls again to live fully. We have to open up all the places we have shut down, or we will never have access to all the feelings we want and deserve to experience. Vulnerability actually means having a huge amount of courage to let yourself be seen.

Myth 2: I Don't Do Vulnerability

Every time you choose to engage in life by having an honest conversation, offering your help, or acting as a good listener, you are being vulnerable. When you show up in your own life or someone else's and engage yourself, that is also vulnerability.

Vulnerability is hard if there is a worthiness crisis going on. But showing up in your life requires vulnerability on your part. Regardless of your socialization patterns or how scared you are to look behind your beliefs and discover your emotions or feelings, the way to stop chronic dieting and compulsive eating is to feel and share your emotions instead of hiding and numb them. Emotional eaters can find it difficult to become vulnerable because we feel that our worthiness is on the line.

But worthiness is a birthright for everyone. We each have the right to be silly, foolish, or imperfect and can be loved even more for that. Brokenness is learned, not innate. I believe that we need to engage in friendships and partnerships where we can be who we really are and not who we thing we are supposed to be. Being vulnerable and imperfectly perfect is a birthright, not a privilege. As Brené Brown once said that when it comes to vulnerability, "It is the first thing I look for in you, but it is the last thing I want you to see in me. In you it is courage; in me it is an inadequacy. In you it's strength and lovability; in me it's shame." In other words, most of the time when we see people being vulnerable, we think it's courage. But when we think about vulnerability in ourselves, we think of it as weakness. It's time to change and show up in your life. That's the only way to have a real life—not just a pretended one or an imagined one, but a well-lived one.

Women and girls struggling with shame and insecurity, chronic dieting, and chronic weight fluctuation have a tendency to cover up their emotions to numb their feelings when they feel vulnerable. So we instead armor up against vulnerability and use numbing and binging. And then we experience many of the self-conscious feelings like guilt, shame, embarrassment, and humiliation. Vulnerability is the birthplace of understanding who you are and what you need and want in your life to be truly happy. Getting over compulsive eating requires becoming vulnerable and experiencing your emotions. Put another way, in order to feel what you need, you must become vulnerable.

Fragmented society and the breakdown of family structures can make it difficult for anyone to understand the universal truth that our worthiness don't depend on our career, money, fame, body weight, shape, or economic status.

Reestablishing a true connection to our self-worth is much needed for anyone who has compulsive behavior of any kind.

We all have a mental list about our prerequisites for worthiness, unfortunately. These can be different for everybody. What's on your list? Have you ever thought about it this way? You might say that you have pretty high self-esteem, so you would assume that's a straight line to a strong sense of worthiness. However, that's often not true in reality.

A lot of times, people with sufficient self-esteem still struggle with chronic dieting, compulsive eating, or weight fluctuations. People at the top of their game can be found on this list as well. Folks with high self-esteem often think that their self-worth is based on performance or appearance. So, who do they become if they lose their job or their looks?

The mainstream idea is that self-esteem is a great building block to grow self-worth. When I ask people about self-esteem, they think about it in relation to their successes or failures. We were told that if we build self-esteem, we would feel much better about ourselves and have a strong sense of self-worth. But there is a huge difference between self-esteem and self-worth.

Self-esteem is based on what we do, how people see us, what we think about ourselves, and how we are doing compared to others. Self-esteem, in contrast, has to do with our strength and limitations. Self-worth is not about who you are or what you do or have; it's about how you treat yourself regardless. Self-worth has to do with whether you respect or have a favorable opinion of yourself.

I am not saying that low self-esteem isn't the reason for body image insecurity, weight struggles, or compulsive eating behaviors; it can absolutely affect you. I am suggesting that regardless of whether you have low or high self-esteem, that's only part of the story in relation to how much you love and accept yourself. When there is a weight struggle and troubled relationship with food, there is always body image insecurity as well, and this goes back to fighting for your worthiness. When you have high self-esteem, you can still experience low self-worth and self-love. This eventually shows up in your eating behaviors and weight struggles.

Eleanor Roosevelt once said, "No one can make you feeling inferior without your consent." Her statement is quite relevant to the topic of this chapter.

When I was studying holistic nutrition, emotional, mental, and spiritual health was part of the curriculum in addition to nutrition and food. However, I never expected that mental and emotional health were going to be such a huge part of my professional life.

An ongoing struggle with your weight or negative body image is very much connected to mental health. Overcoming core beliefs or limiting beliefs often comes up in relation to those who feel unworthy of love, unacceptable, unlovable, and generally unacceptable. Being upset or obsessed with your body to feel likeable by others and to accept yourself come from negative beliefs about yourself, heavily influenced by cultural messages. TV, magazines, and other forms of media target women and girls with the message that we are not worthy of love unless we meet the super thin standard for attractiveness.

Core beliefs are so deeply rooted in our mind that it takes time to change them. But before that comes awareness and critical thinking. Emotional and mental challenges can show up in your life by feelings of insecurity, uncertainty, anxiety, dependency on others, perfectionism, and so on. By shedding light on distorted thought patterns and identifying ways to change them, people often begin to feel better immediately. I sure did.

When you check in with yourself more often, it will get easier to identify and express your emotions if you have a sense of good self-worth and deserving.

Experiencing feelings of being flawed or insufficient is a product of living in modern society. Whether you picked up your insecurities from within your family environment or outside of it, shame makes it difficult to embrace who you are and have a strong sense of self-worth.

Because of the cultural standards we encounter every day, we are convinced that weight is one of the best indicators of our value in society. Being skinny seems more important than being smart and talented. We are worried and stressed out, and if we stop striving to be skinny, we panic. However, panic can feel good; it makes us feel that we can somehow lose the weight if we keep panicking. It is very common to do that rather than facing our struggle with weight. If we hide behind panicking as the solution for weight loss, it is like saying that we are not good enough the way we are—we are flawed. We deny our self-worth, and we believe we can only be happy with a specific number on a scale. Unrealistic cultural standards and demands get in the way of accepting ourselves, and our struggle for worthiness manifests itself in controlling our weight, appetite, and body.

But you can't find or feel your self-worth outside of you. It is something you must cultivate inside yourself deliberately. You are able to evaluate it, develop it, or manage it. When emotional well-being is nowhere to be found, it is partially because of the way you think about yourself. When your thoughts don't serve you, your behaviors can dramatically increase your misalignment. When this happens, you will likely develop some psychological behavior patterns such as a disease to please, fear of failure or rejection, perfection syndrome, procrastination, poor boundary setting with others, and more. These habitual behaviors can ultimately drive you to have compulsive behaviors like shopping, zoning out on TV, numbing out on food, or gambling.

When you are on the path of personal development and growth, you will feel vulnerable. You feel this way because of the fears or traumas you experienced in your past. Limiting beliefs always go back to an incident that happened previously, and now the experience plays upon your present patterns of thinking and feeling. Modern society also encourages you to stand out from others and make a name for yourself. This wouldn't be a problem if culture didn't also teach you to base your self-worth on the success of these things. Take the steps described in the following section to break this unhealthy pattern.

Evaluate what you were taught about self-worth when you were growing up. Were you supposed to behave or dress a certain way to feel worthy? Were you told that you had less worth because of certain outcomes of your duties? Ask yourself these questions and write out your beliefs. Since our society places more value on self-esteem than on self-worth, it is really helpful to see what you learned about self-worth. Next, evaluate the list you wrote. One of the easiest ways to do this is to see if your self-talk reflects what you believe to be true about yourself. Identify and hold onto the beliefs that serve you or feel right to you, and find out what needs to be tweaked or removed.

If you discover any beliefs or reactions to an event that don't serve you but still provide an emotional charge, it means the belief, event, or experience hasn't been processed yet. It might be hard to recognize your limiting beliefs because they feel true to you. When you were young, you couldn't choose the basis of your self-worth; your caregivers defined it, and now your mind chatter repeats it. Your self-talk is a reflection of your deeper beliefs. Don't expect to have a strong sense of self-worth overnight, especially if you have been hard on yourself for a while.

Get clear on what your self-talk says with regard to each belief you hold on to. If any of the messages are not supportive, you need to improve them. If you believe that it is your birthright to experience happiness, joy, fulfillment, and being genuine, then you can trust yourself. To really understand your relationship with food, you have to understand your relationship with life. Most of us restrict food to trust ourselves around it.

Our emotional appetite will only decrease when we are emotionally full.

Doing only what you are told to do also means you don't trust yourself. You likely picked up messages from your environment that said you are only as good as your body looks, but let me ask you this: Do you really want to let yourself feel damaged or insufficient based on the size of your body? Does this really make sense?

I understand that we live in a world where a first impression is everything, and there are some people who have the ideal body that present society idolizes. It might be easer for them to get things, but in real life, people remember how you make them feel more than they remember how you look or what you say, as Maya Angelou reminds us.

Living your life fully is not about what you do or don't have. Beliefs that feel good to you may result in good things, but if you attain money, fame, or a nice car by restricting yourself from things you believe so that you feel worthy, and if your self-talk is critical, you will still feel miserable when you get want you want.

This is also true with weight loss or weight management. Pushing yourself, restricting yourself, or allowing critical self-talk might give you the body you want, but in the end, you will not like yourself more. However if the outcome of self-compassion, self-love, and self-worth is losing weight, you will not only keep the weight off but also be truly happy with your new body from the inside. While you were working toward that goal, you also grew a sense of love and worthiness toward yourself.

Myth 3: We Can Do It Alone

Our inner desires to love, to be loved, and to belong can't be fulfilled unless we engage and interact with others. Unfortunately the U.S. culture is based on individualism and the motto, "I can do it alone."

Wanting to do it alone relates to the thought pattern of how we perceive getting vulnerable with others because it requires putting down our guard regardless of knowing the outcome. I believe we are not only afraid of being seen but also afraid of being rejected for not being good enough when we are seen. But real love and belonging can only exist when we love people not despite what they show when they're vulnerable but because of it.

When you decide to disengage from feelings and emotions through not practicing vulnerability, you are choosing to disengage from your life. You refuse to discover what makes you alive. Instead of sticking with willpower to diet or obsess over food, you want to find out who you are and how your life would look if you didn't have this preoccupation.

115

As mentioned previously, the first step to overcoming compulsive eating of any forms is to choose to experience your feelings instead of eating them.

Reconnect With the Feelings You Have

If you don't become aware of your feelings, you won't know what you are creating in your life. Emotions are a type of energy in the body, and if you suppress them, they get trapped in your body, and this can show up in the form of health problems.

To practice experiencing your feelings instead of eating them, ask yourself these two questions:

- What do I feel?
- How do I feel?

Allow yourself ninety seconds to engage and process the feeling. This allows you to create a space between the feeling and the reaction.

I understand that you probably want to avoid your feelings, so instead of being present with them, you usually deliberately change the emotions you feel, and your method of change is food. From now on, I invite you to move toward those emotions instead of avoiding them. You run away from your feelings because you think they will destroy you. But if notice and experience them, the feelings will transform overtime. It is not the feelings that hurt so much but the stories you tell yourself about them. You take what you have experienced so far in life and form belief systems out it, and then the stories you attach to your feelings become your reality.

Your feelings are a perceptive state of consciousness. When you experience emotions, you in essence perceive your physiological reaction to your thoughts. And your thoughts dictate your vibrations. In essence, you are not really your body. Your body is like everybody else's in the universe: It is just energy in vibration. Your emotions perceive your body's translation of this vibration. Fortunately, you can change your feelings if you can stop being resistant to them. Trying to push down your feelings or avoid them by eating is a form of resistance, for example. And you can choose to release the resistance and go in the direction of your feelings.

When you become mindful, you understand that your emotions can overtake your mind, making you feel overwhelmed and out of control. If you observe a feeling that you experience and let yourself be conscious of it, you can notice your feelings changing by themselves.

Acceptance represents being able to stay with how you feel and ride out the urge (craving) until it is gone. It is about standing back and observing what's happening without overidentifying with your thoughts and feelings or acting on them. It means not being on automatic pilot. It involves a breathing exercise. And it is an approach that believes the more you give in to cravings, the more you reinforce their power. Instead, you can ride the wave of a craving, using your breath as a metaphorical surfboard.

The term "urge surfing" refers to a technique attributed to psychologist Alan Marlatt, Ph.D. It basically means surfing on the physical sensations in your body. Feelings always come and go; they never stay the same, and by looking at urges like waves, we see that they rise in intensity, peak, and eventually crash. Surfing the urge when you want to binge involves curiosity to know what you feel. For example, do you feel scared, happy, anxious, stressed out, or depressed? Up until this point, you have been trying to keep your feelings away to temporarily feel safe.

Surfing the urge of cravings is not trying to fix ourselves. It is an attempt to understand who we are in the part of us that feels. In other words, we are trying to discover what was placed in our minds when we were young and in school and who we take ourselves to be based on what we picked up from our environment. Remember, it is not the feeling that is hard to deal with but the belief we attach to it.

When you can allow yourself to be present in your feelings but not sink into them, you have a chance to understand who you are.

When you truly understand that your task is not to pick up on things that are bad in you and fix them but instead to connect the dots and take responsibility to see what might have to be shifted or perceived differently, you are on your way to real happiness. When you can believe that not everything you thought about yourself was true, you are ready to transform your life and ultimately your body. When you can be aware of what you think and feel like an observer without drowning in them, it is like being able to connect with your feelings instead of relating to them distantly.

This relates to the idea I quoted earlier from Gary Zukav's work. When you are ready to question and therefore feel what you feel— anger, sadness, happiness, joy, or fear—with kindness, curiosity, and compassion instead of judgment, rejection, and numbing emotions with food, you stand at the door containing answers for all your issues with dieting, emotional eating, and your body.

You can trace your present feelings back to the moments you first felt them. And revealing your feelings is the key to revealing the beliefs you are holding on to, based on your experiences. Remember, the stories you tell yourself about moments in the past and the feelings that come from them operate on a subconscious level.

When you start practicing this method, you will likely have many slipups. If you can find a little part of you willing to do this exercise, keep going. I've become very good at it over time, but it took me a lot of practice. But as rewriting neural pathways is possible, you will change your routine and give in to fewer cravings than before. Think about it this way: Whatever you repeat and focus on doing gets stronger, and anything you don't practice gets weaker. Surfing the urge is a choice. Being on autopilot is a choice. Food cravings can hit you suddenly, but they also fade away at some point. Think about a natural tide. The biggest waves look dangerous and scary, but at some point they quiet down and become harmless.

Your job is to follow the ways your feelings change and examine the new feelings as they change. Breathe into that new feeling, and move into it and through it consciously. Let yourself be immersed in your feelings but not so much that you sink in them or overidentify with them, as mentioned previously.

Viktor E. Frankl, an Austrian neurologist and psychiatrist, said, "Between stimulus and response there is a space. In that space is our power to choose our response. In our response lies our growth and our freedom." The method described above is closely related to Frankl's statement.

It is like you create space between your thoughts and your reaction. As previously mentioned, feelings are sensations in your body, but the stories you create about them are the reactions of your beliefs. While surfing an urge, your mind may wander to a story that you are telling yourself. When this happens, come back and feel anything that comes up. When you can stay with the sensation of your feelings, you will see as an energy form within your body; it will transform over and over into different feelings until you feel a positive sensation, and then there are no more layers covering your true essence.

This is your chance to explore what you feel and where you sense it. Does your feeling have a shape, texture, temperature, or color? Where do you feel it? Is it in your chest, heart, head, legs, or arms? Do you feel vibration in your stomach or pulsing in your chest? Give your feelings some room. How old do the sensations make you feel? Remember, feelings are sensations in your body, but thoughts about these sensations are beliefs you formed based on your experience. If you can't stand your feelings and want to eat compulsively, that's also a reaction to a sensation that you associate with emotions. With certain feelings, you shut yourself down with food to ease the experience. That's why I recommend that you detach yourself from the beliefs connected to feelings, not from the feelings themselves.

As discussed previously, emotional eaters often want to disconnect and numb themselves with food because of the social conditioning that stigmatizes sharing feelings and emotions. We become fearful of having them at all. However, by resisting feelings rather than being aware of them, we disown our inner GPS systems and get cut off from knowing what's best for us. This ultimately shows up in how we relate to life, to friends, or to food. A compulsive eater that wishes to change has no choice but to feel his or her feelings instead of eating them.

Your job in this step is to draw in a deep breath through your nose and breathe out through your mouth. What are the texture and color of the feelings in your body? Does anything feel tight? Take more deep breaths and release the feeling as you breathe out. You will feel much lighter and relieved; it is like being less at war with yourself. You need to breathe, reconnect, and let go.

It is okay if it is hard at first; you might not know what you feel or what to do. You are on the path of trying to release what's blocking your awareness.

On a moment-by-moment basis, reconnect with a feeling when you are in the middle of chaos, and say the following silently or out loud:

"Help me to release the fear of ..." Fill in the blank, and then breathe in and out. By doing this, you will change your energy and ultimately your feelings and emotions as well.

Self-Care Skill Four: Practice Self-Soothing without Eating

If you were taught how to create a nurturing, supportive, calming, and reassuring inner world, most likely your ability to self-soothe yourself when needed is very high.

At its core, self-soothing means that you are able to establish an emotional independency apart from others. You are able to cope with difficult situations by self-soothing and restore your emotional balance. You can learn this skill at any age. However, if you get stuck in emotions, whether pleasant or unpleasant, and have no way to process them, you are more likely to use coping mechanisms such as binging or overeating. It is not the worst thing to do, but it gets in the way of managing your weight and living with inner peace.

Feeling resistant to self-soothing can be a sign that you are not yet ready for adult self-care. It takes practice. When you are anxious or stressed out, it is often hard to think about self-soothing without eating because you can't think clearly.

Every time compulsive, absentminded eating shows up in your life, you can start creating new habits to overcome it. We must take steps to overcome self-soothing with food, as it has become so ingrained. Adult self-care involves distraction (from the compulsion), emotional release, surfing the urge, and solving the reason you want to overeat. Let's look at each of these methods separately.

1. Distraction

Adult self-soothing behaviors include centering or grounding yourself, and they are a set of simple tools to help you detach from emotional or mental disturbance, imbalance, or pain.

Binging on food or overeating is a form of distraction when you are vulnerable to your emotions and flooded with feelings you can't handle. You need a time out. You want to leave your significant other, so you binge. Happy emotions can take you down the road of emotional eating as well.

The key to place a healthier distraction when you are out of emotional balance is to find something compelling enough to take your thoughts away from binging or overeating. The goal is to stimulate your mind or body to take your mind off of compulsive eating. You can't just stare at a wall. You need to get out of an emotional loop. You have to do this each time you get the craving.

Putting more distractions in place doesn't solve the problem that triggered your eating, but it will change your perception that you can't do anything but eat to soothe yourself. You need to create a habit change that requires patience and discipline.

Following are some ideas for distraction that you can use. What you choose to do can vary depending on where you are when you get the craving.

- Watch your favorite show on TV.
- Use the Internet or read a book.
- Chew on something like gum, straw, a toothpick, or cinnamon sticks.
- Play games on your phone as a focused activity.
- Flip through some magazines you like or books that have lots of pictures. Don't think too deeply. Just turn the pages and enjoy it.
- Think of something funny to jolt yourself out of your present mood. Watch something that makes you smile. For example, I like to watch *The Ellen DeGeneres Show*.
- Make a playlist beforehand and listen to any kind of music you find stimulating or calming to change the mood you are in.

Using distraction only works as an immediate Band-Aid solution. No more and no less. It doesn't solve the underlying issue driving your compulsive eating. When you are tired of feeling powerless and you don't want to be the victim of your thoughts or emotions, you will choose something instead of distraction. However, it is best not to disconnect from yourself by finding another compulsive practice as a substitute for your compulsive eating. When you stop wanting to go from one numbing behavior to the next, you are ready to practice self-soothing, and is a great sign that you are ready to take responsibility for your life. But distracting yourself from eating is the first step in your transformation.

Action Step:

Create a list of things that work to distract you from food thoughts and compulsive eating.

2. Emotional Release

As mentioned previously, emotional eaters like to eat their feelings instead of feeling them. Your menu of emotional management can only get better when you are able to release the feelings in your body. Many times, it is easy to get stuck on emotions we feel familiar with because we are used to them, but it doesn't mean they still add benefit to our life. But the familiarity makes it feel safe, even if it doesn't feel good.

Emotional freedom can only happen when you are able to release the energy in the form of these feelings that keep you stuck. Holding onto emotions will keep you in a loop where your compulsive activity—whether that shows up in emotional eating, watching TV for hours without paying attention, or surfing the Internet without feeling replenished—ultimately directs you to zone out of life. Whether you are able to solve the issue that makes you want to overeat or not, releasing feelings will help you restore your emotional balance and stop you from wanting to eat compulsively.

Conscious complaining is one way to carry out this therapeutic emotional release. Try journaling or complaining out loud when no one is around. You can swear the hell out of your issue. A good cry never hurt either.

Physical activity is great for releasing energy and feelings. Do a high-intensity exercise for thirty seconds or a minute, such as burpees, push-ups, squat jumps, high knees, or anything that your physical ability allows.

Let Go of the Emotional Weight

What emotional weight are you carrying around? What kind of psychological traumas and emotional injuries have you suffered? Where is your emotional flow blocked?

- Look at the following words and phrases.

- Read them carefully a couple of times.
- Allow yourself to connect and identify with the words and what they mean. Let your mind wander around situations as memories and painful experiences come up.

abandonment	unexpressed emotions
attack	burden
separation	unfulfilled
loneliness	unforgiveness
neglect	laziness
injustice	lack of protection
dishonesty	fear of uncertainty
pressure	low self-worth
arrogance	shame
selfishness	exhaustion
rejection	pride
embarrassment	guilt
anger	fear
jealousy	heartbreak
stress	judgment
weight stigma	low self-esteem
body shame	responsibility
greed	

- Now grab a pen and paper.
- Let your emotions and feelings guide you as your thoughts flow onto the paper.
- Write down each word from the list that speaks to you and ask yourself what experience, thought, and emotion the world reflects back to you. What happened to you in the situation? Be as detailed as you can. You can go back and forth between the phrases with no particular order. Spend as much as time as you need on this task. Don't judge yourself. Simply show up in your life. This will allow you to stop fighting for your worthiness.

When you give yourself permission to feel the pain you m.
have denied for so long, it will begin to leave.

- You are welcome to add words not on the list if they come to you and write down your feelings about them.
- Follow this exercise only if you can do it without forcing it. You are working on the inside by opening up to feeling, not from the outside by pushing things on yourself that you don't want to or aren't ready to feel.

Action Step:

Create a list of things that work to release your emotions and stop you from thoughts about food and compulsive eating.

3. Feel Your Feelings by Surfing the Urge

Processing your emotions and feelings sounds like a great idea, but you wouldn't be reading this book if you knew how to do it.

Before you give yourself a hard time, wondering why you can't sit and stay with your emotions or why it's not easy to accept the situations that trigger your emotional eating, know that it's not your fault. The ability to drop the resistance and understand that this is the way things are, bringing your attention to the present moment and accepting the feeling you are swimming in, doesn't come naturally to humans.

Why can't we turn toward the sensation that we experience when we are out of balance emotionally—upset, sad, happy, or anxious—and stay with those sensations? Bruce Tift, psychotherapist, calls this a "counterinstinctual move." He says the practice of sanity is actually counterinstinctual. This may be very helpful for you to hear.

When Bruce Tift interviewed Tami Simon for The Self-Acceptance Project in 2013, they talked about why growth and self-discovery is so hard. "When we feel all stirred up inside and panicky, or when our stomach turns like a mixer, the counterinstinctual move is go out and take a jog, call a friend, or eat cookies to do something to get out immediately. It hurts—it sucks—and we just want to do ~~the~~ paths of growth and self-acceptance to experience those ~~actually hang out with them are counterinstinctual. It is~~ ~~similarly~~ counterinstinctual to breath into the feelings, being aware that we are checking e-mails constantly, watching TV, or standing in front of the fridge to avoid processing those feelings. Ask yourself, "Can I now do the counterinstinctual thing and be with those painful sensations? That's self-acceptance. It means you are accepting and embracing what's happening right now, not turning away from it. Notice the awareness, and then tolerate the intensity of how yucky the anxiety, terror, or panic feels. Can you sit like you are in a fire and burn?"

This requires you to step back from the thinking self and toward the feeling self. When emotions are expressed instead of suppressed, that's where the real magic happens for binge eaters.

You can use this exercise when you have the sudden urge to eat. Distracting yourself in an attempt to run away from your cravings is no different than trying to run away from your problems. They will be there after you stop running. As discussed in an earlier section, urges are like waves: they Arise, reach a peak, and then fall and pass. Allow yourself to see the urge coming, feel it rise, and then watch it peak and fall.

This exercise is about stopping and noticing that you have a desire to eat. Check whether you notice any physical hunger in yourself. When you understand that you are not physically hungry but all you can think about is food, you know it is emotional. After you notice you have a desire to eat, get away from all food if you can. You don't want to smell it, see it, or touch it.

Notice that something has happened to you that may have changed your mood. Maybe you are feeling something related to a memory or someone did or said something to you recently.

Observe your breath, where your mind wanders, and what feelings you feel that make you want to disappear.

Let's focus on your breath. While you notice your breath, sit down, stand in one place, or walk around. What is your breath like? Is it shallow, deep, calm, steady, or quick? Take a few long deep breaths in and out. Don't try to adjust your breath; just watch it. Breathe in and out at your own pace. Is your breathing rapid? Or does it remain long and slow?

Now, notice your thoughts. Don't criticize them, fight them, or try to change them; just observe them. Your thoughts will most likely demand to be heard. And you will likely think about the urge to eat. Let those thoughts enter your mind. Let that urge come over you. Feel it, and let it wash over you. Notice your thoughts as they eventually leave and evolve into new thoughts. Look at this urge again. Don't judge it.

Think about a surfboard and the waves. Notice how much your mind wanders. Waves come and go. The intensity of the cravings will also come and go.

Are you still there? Congratulations. You have just made it to the other side of the wave.

Now, let's check on how your body feels. Where do you feel the physical sensations of your feelings at this moment? Are they in your head, stomach, shoulders, chest, or back? Notice whether you feel one particular feeling or many at the same time.

Now, let's come back to your breath again. Focus on breathing in and out. Don't worry about the rate; do what feels natural.

Now, focus on your body again. Feel the urge as it comes over your physical form. If your feelings could talk, what they would say? Try to describe what you feel. If you can't do this, try to identify the part of your body in which you feel the cravings are coming from. Study the sensations.

Do you know notice anything changing as you breathe? Continue focusing on different parts of your body as you study the sensations and cravings. Become interested and willing to learn more about it. You are practicing curiosity.

As you notice what's happening with your urges, do you see how they increase and decrease? Just like the waves in the ocean, there are peaks and valleys.

Now, let's focus on your feelings again. Surf them like you would surf the waves in an ocean. What do you feel? Where do you feel it?

Breathe in and out at your own space. As you take the time to do this, eventually the urges fully transform as you monitor them. Stay relaxed and focused. Breathe in and out and repeat.

If you still feel the craving, take your mind off your breath and focus on the urge again. Describe the urge. Where is it coming from? Where do you feel it in your body? Stay focused and study it. You are curious; you want to be with the feeling.

Now, breathe in and out again. Try to measure the level of the urge. Has it gotten stronger or decreased?

Tell yourself, "I will feel these feelings a little longer, and if they get too hard to feel, I have the option to eat." Allow yourself to feel what's happening in your body. Your feelings are waiting for you. They naturally come and go. Wanting them to go away remains the same.

At this point, if your urges are still strong, you have two choices: You can give in and eat something you desperately want to, or you can keep going and surf the urge a little longer.

You know that food will not solve anything permanently. But it takes practice to let go of this habit. You are doing great. Just keep practicing regardless of what you decide in a particular instance, and you will get increasingly better at surfing the urge.

When you are able to surf the urge, it proves that you don't want to disown your body. You no longer want to stuff your body with food because your thoughts and emotions influence you to do that. Furthermore, surfing the urge shows that you truly understand that when you are done eating, the problem will still be there, and you just added to the problem by adding weight to your waistline. You understand that if right now, without looking perfect or having solved all of your issues, you can still get back on your feet without numbing, your life will unfold in front of you. When you no longer believe your body must look a certain way or you must own certain things, you accept that moving through your emotions and feelings rather than stuffing them down is the only way to have a real life.

Never think you have to excuse yourself for feeling a certain way. Walk into your life and own your story. When you are used to experiencing your feelings instead of eating them, your weight will no longer be an excuse to avoid your real life and issues. So, when you look back on this time in several decades, you can say that you not only lived through your life experiences but also that you felt every second of them.

Something happens every time you accept your feelings. It feels like relief. Accepting your feelings means you are willing to sense them instead of resisting them.

Do your feelings make you cold or hot? Sense the texture of a feeling. Imagine its shape or color. This allows you to transform the energy (feeling) that lives inside of you and turn it into a mental picture. Your mind and imagination act as the silver bullet you've been looking for.

Staying with your feelings in the present helps anchor you to the present moment and keeps you from contemplating the past or worrying about the future. Remember, emotional pain is a feeling. Don't over identify with it, as it is not who you are. When you get caught up in pain, it feels like your only reality, and it seems like it will never go away. However, it is only a part of your experience in the present moment; emotions always come and go. Understanding and expressing emotions in different situations is the elixir against binging and weight gain. This means we need to get vulnerable and get in touch with ourselves by listening to how we feel and not what we think.

Surfing the urge and flowing with your emotions requires one thing: You need to show up for your feelings. Promise yourself that you will show up even if you are scared or shaking. This will become more challenging before it gets better. All of the feelings you have been numbing for so long are current and present. They might feel like butterflies in your stomach or tingling at first. Then you might sense all the feelings you have been covering up like guilt, shame, uncertainty, hopelessness, and so on. This can feel like somebody hitting your chest hard. Your mind always wanders to the past in the form of you could have or should have done or to the future with what ifs. But real human beings return to the present and experience their feelings of the moment.

I am the same person as when I was sixteen years old, the time period when I felt excited, scared, or worried all the time and started to numb my feelings through eating. I still have a lot of emotional ups and downs, every day, all day. But instead of believing that I am wrong or something is wrong with me, I accept this part of myself, and no one can tell me otherwise. This is part of the human experience.

I know that running for the exit won't do any good in my life. I have been there too many times. The problem will stay inside of me and come up later. I used to numb myself, zone out, and hide how I felt, but now I share how I feel. That's the only difference.

Feelings generally last for about a minute, but if you keep replaying them over and over, it's hard to find inner peace. Come back to the present moment and say, "All I have is the present moment. And right now, I am just fine."

4. Solving the Why

Try to solve the root cause creating the emotions and feelings that trigger your emotional eating. Behind every compulsive behavior, there

is a trigger. Your job is to puzzle out what causes yo
emotional balance and makes you want to eat.

Many times, the thoughts and feelings that evoke the
trigger eating compulsively arise when we compare them to an idea
regarding what we are supposed to be, to have, or to do. And if they
don't fit, we get out of balance.

Ask yourself the following questions before you reach for food to
numb your feelings:

- If I weren't thinking about food, what would I be thinking
  about?
- What I am looking for in this food?
- What do I need right now?

Check in with yourself to see whether any of the following are true:

- Someone said something that makes you want to eat.
- Someone did something that makes you want to eat.
- You have a strong feeling.

Also, ask these questions after you binge or overeat:

- What was I thinking about immediately before I suddenly
  wanted to binge?
- What happened immediately before I suddenly started to think
  about food?
- Where was I?
- Who I was talking to?
- Did someone say something?
- Did someone do something?

Getting into the habit of looking for answers, whether you actually
eat or not, creates the opportunity to have light-bulb moments and
become aware of what fuels your emotional eating. That's when the real
work begins. When you feel fear of any kind, you can find the medicine

your pain. When you get some answers, brainstorm possible action steps and take immediate action.

Remember, until the pain of remaining in the situation is more than making the change, you will keep choosing emotional eating.

Even if you didn't grow up with the ability to nurture yourself, you can learn to have the ability at any stage of life, as mentioned previously. Your inner nurturer provides a connection to your core self—the voice inside of you that can be compassionate, loving, supporting, and understanding. Some people are luckier than others and develop this nurturing voice while they're growing up. Either their caregivers model it, or they are born with more awareness of what's going on outside of them. But most of us who have issues with compulsive behaviors need to learn our way there.

Remember that the alliance you form between your mind chatter and your inner nurturer is ultimately the turning point to getting your needs met. Therefore, maintaining an ongoing connection with your inner nurturer is important.

Being able to pinpoint the emotion and the reason you want to numb out can ease your mind and help you think about the action steps to solve the issue that triggered emotional eating.

As suggested earlier in this chapter, try to take mental notes about what was happening before you decided to binge. What did you do? Where were you? Who said or did what? Notice how you felt and reacted. Did you feel scared, uncertain, or anxious? Notice if your binging is a way of processing something you can't express directly. Additionally, observe whether your binging makes you disconnect from your body. Did you feel a sense of calm or security while you were eating? How did food make you feel?

Although this book aims to give you practical suggestions and solutions for discovering the reasons you emotionally eat, I can't tell you that having the tools will give you the ultimate solution. There is no such a thing in emotional eating. Like with any compulsive behavior, overcoming emotional eating takes practice. There is no such thing as failure, but there are a lot of learning curves in the process.

Compulsive eating can be the product of your emotional, mental, or spiritual state. If you are out of alignment in any of these areas, compulsive eating takes the edge off a feeling you can't feel with food. Connecting with yourself via the questions I gave you above can help you to discover what you are truly hungry for.

You may also want to evaluate your life in regard to the following areas:

- Being listened to
- Participating in fun group activities
- Spending time with friends
- Exercising
- Having unplugged time
- Having downtime
- Having creative time
- Having a sense of accomplishment
- Receiving physical touch, hugs, or sex
- Enjoying stimulating conversation
- Having spiritual time
- Laughing
- Playing or listening to music
- Spending time outdoors
- Feeling a sense of belonging
- Spending time without the need to accomplish anything
- Sleeping
- Handling stress

The methods of using distractions, surfing the urge, and learning about the reasons for your behavior are not meant to cause you guilt or shame. Some days you will be better at practicing than others. This part of the book is focused on discovering the real you and learning about yourself. Be as gentle and compassionate toward yourself as you would be with someone whom you love very much.

If you feel overwhelmed by your emotions and feelings, it can be a sign that certain skills might need sharpening. You will feel raw when you are vulnerable, but as you practice self-connection, it gets better and easier with time. If you feel too overwhelmed, take a break. Don't push it if you feel too uncomfortable. You can distract yourself at this point in the process. Don't look at it as a sign of weakness. Everything takes practice. Anytime you get an impulse to eat emotionally, don't try to avoid the feeling that triggered the craving. Your mindfulness practice allows you to see the urges like waves.

You always have the option to use distractions, surf the urge, or discover the reason instead of eating. Come up with a toolbox that works for you. At the point when you are not hungry but want to eat to take the edge off a feeling that you can't or don't know how to handle, you always have a choice. You can feel your feelings or them. Never judge yourself, no matter how you choose to deal with your feelings. Judgment closes your heart and creates fear.

The direction you take regarding your mistakes and not feeling good enough creates a decision point in terms of how willing you are to feel your emotions and examine the connected beliefs. Preventing binging or stopping in the moment of binging requires passing through your defense mechanism because wanting to stay present with your unpleasant emotions and feelings is not your default response yet.

Lastly, understanding something intellectually is one thing, and implementing it on a daily basis is another thing. Don't be too hard on yourself when you are aware of your compulsive behavior but can't do anything but eat. The more you deny yourself the option of indulging in your binge, the more difficult it will be to get away from it. What you resist persists. So, let your mind process the information you have learned here. Shift from binging to wanting to distract yourself with something else, surf the urge, and solve the issue behind emotional eating. Change your perception instead of forcing yourself to do what you know intellectually. Pushing requires willpower, and it will never last. There are certain times in your life that you can't figure out the root cause of your emotions and feelings, or you don't have the skills yet that allow you to move through your emotions. Sometimes circumstances put you in a place where you can only think about finding a coping mechanism for your emotional eating. It is not the best thing to do but also not the worst. Acknowledge that you are trying to cope with emotional eating in another way, but if nothing works out, you still have the option to numb out on food. If the feelings are very bad, you know that you can eat. The option needs to be there. If you happen to binge on food, practice slowing down and stopping after a couple of bites to see how you feel, and go from there.

Self-Care Skill Five: Empower Your Soul

Drop into Happiness

Hopefully, you understand now that permanent weight loss is not the key to happiness because you can't make other people responsible for your happiness. That would be an unfair burden on them. When you make your happiness a priority by creating a life you wish you had regardless of how your body looks, eventually your insecurities about your body will no longer be your default response.

Our self-worth is tied to our net worth and to our level of productivity. If we don't feel exhausted at the end of the day, it's like we didn't do enough to feel good about ourselves. We bond over comparing our exhaustion levels at work and at home. However, in countries like Spain, it is okay and even encouraged to take a nap during the day. Can you image the same being true in the United States? I don't think so. Exhaustion is a status symbol.

When we were young, activities that felt good to us, such as singing, playing, and dancing were a normal part of life. We could enjoy a good laugh or downtime, and we played for fun. We had not yet been taught that we needed to be concerned with how we looked and with what others thought of us, we danced and laughed with joy and pleasure. But we were eventually taught through socialization, which becomes a deeply ingrained cultural belief, that it is not okay to play and dance anymore.

Grown-ups need to take life seriously in order to get somewhere in life. Spending time doing purposeless activities because they feel good becomes rare once we are adults. Shame gremlins easily hit us when we engage is something that doesn't necessarily pay the bills. We are afraid that other people will perceive us as selfish if we want to have some me time.

We women and girls are programed that self-sacrifice makes us better and that self-care—including fun and relaxation—makes us selfish and useless. Women and girls are supposed to take care of others.

But what if it is important to feed our soul? When the soul or spirit doesn't get cared for, it begins to die; so does the body. From that point, we seek out distractions like zoning out on TV or eating when we are not hungry. In contrast, when you stand up for yourself and create a life involving joy, fun, laughter, and dance, you will be a better mother, wife, girlfriend, friend, or colleague. You can be "selfish" enough to nourish your soul on a daily basis rather than looking for excuses not to do so. You will not fill up on food to the point of overindulgence or become immersed in your negative self-talk because your soul is deprived. Instead, you will take dance lessons, watch comedies, paint, ride your bicycle for fun, swim, or create something without a specific purpose or agenda.

Thoughts and beliefs as well as feelings and emotions can trigger our problem with food and weight, but our soul the core of who we are is the key to ultimately create change in our lives.

No matter how your body looks right now—large or lean—it is only the current manifestation of your soul. In other words, your body is the result of anything you created that lies within. Our spirit doesn't want to suffer; it is only looking for love and self-expression. Deep down, we all want to be in a state of who we truly are because it feels good.

With mainstream weight-loss programs, although you might see quick results in losing weight, your soul doesn't get nourished. Unless your soul is fed with joy, the yearning for a healthy, fit body is almost impossible to fulfill, because it will always reach for something else as nourishment. And in your case, that will usually be food.

Psychotherapists can help us understand the root causes of the negative thinking that forces us to go on diets to get a better body so that we can love ourselves. They can also help us understand why we develop body fixations and compulsive behaviors around food. This book goes into great detail on emotionally driven dieting or self-injuring patterns with food. With that said, don't wait for a specific moment in your life where you feel that your destructive emotions are gone, allowing you to wake up one morning and find the struggle in the past. That is not how it works.

The real work is to understand that while we are all working on ourselves by overcoming our woundedness, it is essential to add love and joy, which ultimately fill up our souls. If we only focus on figuring out the negative, that is just half of the process. The disease of adulthood is seriousness, so we must seek out joy on a daily basis.

We can be so hung up on nutrition goals, health goals, or fitness goals. It's great to have them, but I invite you to have even bigger goal in your life: engaging in activities that you truly enjoy. You can express yourself and be the empowered version of the real you, because that's what brings ultimate happiness.

Working inward by empowering your soul rather than working out with chronic exercise is the goal. Your body is the manifestation of the work that you do within, as discussed previously.

The bravest thing that you can do is to own what makes you alive and love yourself in the meantime. Knowing you are enough no matter what other people think takes courage. And speaking honestly about who you are and what you desire in a relationship or at work takes courage. Most of the weight you carry around is the result of not being the real you. Your turning point for letting go of emotional weight is in expressing your true self and what brings joy, fun, and contentment in your life. Ask your soul who you really are. What does your soul want to express?

Permanent weight loss doesn't start on the outside but on the inside. Body shape shifting doesn't happen in the visible but first in the invisible. Working in what shapes the body first of all and not working out.

Dance, paint, play, sing, or do something creative, even if you are an adult. Empowering your soul by cultivating what feels good to you will fill up your heart with joy, and you will not need food for emotional nourishment.

Take Action:

Binging and overeating can happen because we feel alone and don't know how to spend time with ourselves. Food relaxes us, and then we feel less lonely. Creating a life where you can enjoy time on your own is something we have to learn. Instead of always taking care of others, we must take responsibility to fill up on things that excite us and things that are fun. Learn what truly lights you up. Following is the list I've created for myself:

- Stay connected. Instead of staying at home to avoid social activities with food, I look for connections, friendships, and spontaneous nights out. My spirit and soul always thank me for that. (This was a hard one for me because I am super introverted, but once I am out with people I like, I enjoy my time, and I am emotionally recharged after that.)
- Visit a bookstore to browse books. I look for things that interest me and sit down with a drink. I also enjoy the ambiance of the bookstore.
- Movie night out is a regular item on my list. Whether alone or with somebody, it is great for adding fun into my life.
- Connect with nature. Walking or hiking gives me peace of mind, no matter what is going on in my life.
- Phone dates with friends or family members.
- People watching makes me feel connected.
- Listen to podcasts and relate to something inspirational.

- Create something for myself or for others. Creative work makes me feel grounded. As I focus on the creation, I get out of my mind and tap into timeless eternity.
- Communicate with others. Whether I work from home or surrounded by a lot of people, communicating with friends and family throughout the day about plans and ideas feels comforting to me. We humans are wired for connection, whether introvert or extrovert.
- I search for the type of music I love, and I listen to it often. Music has the power to shift emotions. It is a great way to feel connected to myself.
- I dance even though I am an adult. Dance is full-body vulnerability. It is not about how well I can dance but how much I can get lost in the rhythm of the music. I had to relearn that happiness can be measured by how much dance is present in someone's life.

Part IV
Building a New Home in Your Body

Get into Self-Acceptance

"How much we know ourselves is extremely important but how we treat ourselves is the most important." Brené Brown.

As mentioned previously, getting the perfect body is not going to fix anything because that's not the root cause of your issues.

Weight struggles, lack of body acceptance, and body hate are the products of your internal struggle of not feeling good enough. They are not the cause. You criticize and judge your body because you think that's what stops you from getting the life you want, but your lack of self-love and self-acceptance and the worthiness crisis is underneath your weight struggle.

The moment you are able to look at your unbalanced state as a product of your emotional, mental, and spiritual instability and communicate via love instead of fear, you will end up with an ideal body that you always dreamed of. A shift in perception is the key to get over chronic dieting and compulsive eating and be successful in long-term weight management.

Developing self-acceptance is an individual process. You can't look to anyone else to create it for you. Some people were raised by parents who helped them develop self-nurturing skills. Some parents reflect the ideas of true self-worth. But the majority of us need to work our way there.

The process of obtaining self-acceptance and feeling a sense of self-love and self-worth, no matter what, is accessible to anybody. But you have to make different choices ever-single day than you did so far. Making the right choices for yourself is the most important thing. Managing your weight successfully and not experiencing the yo-yo effect while leaving behind your compulsive eating patterns or body image insecurities is about embracing who you are behind your emotions and feelings.

Body image issues are not related to how you look. Your body image only gets better when you can think about yourself as beautiful, confident, and good enough. If you got the perfect body somehow but didn't change how you feel or treat yourself, your body image in your mind will not change. You can get compliments, but if you don't think you are worthy and special, then body acceptance can't happen. Don't think that self-love and self-acceptance is about liking your abs or your butt. This is shallow compared to real self-love.

Self-love is therefore the solution to body image insecurities and body hate.

When you change from the inside, you will see your body in a new light. When you have a big enough reason to take care of yourself, you will be able to start working on yourself first.

I love the concept of self-acceptance, which comes from having a sense of self-worth and self-love. But if you don't like your body, change it. If you hate your body, transform it. If you don't like something about your butt, shoulders, or abs, and it is changeable, change your form.

But if you dislike your body to the extent that you put your self-worth on line and you can't love yourself because of it, you need to work on the inside as well. You might go into training because of aesthetics, but you need to address the real reason behind your lack of love for your body.

How many times have you met a woman who looked picture perfect, but you could tell from the way she talked about herself that she didn't really like herself. This person might be you. This shows how body image issues are more than just aesthetics.

Action Steps:

Write down why you would invest in your personal growth. Why would you even bother to spend time figuring out your issues regarding your body image insecurity? Once you nail them down, you can see why it is worth working on your issues.

Self-Love Takes Practice

Bell Hooks said, "Practicing love and belonging to begin by always thinking of love as an action rather than a feeling is one way is which anyone using the word in this manner automatically assumes accountability and responsibility."

This quote inspires me to think about self-love and self-worth in the same way. Neither has anything to do with what you do, what you have, or who you are. It is about how you treat yourself. Arriving at self-worth and self-love is possible. Feeling a deep sense of love and belonging doesn't only mean the capacity to love other people; it also means you believe that you are loveable the way you are. In relationships, when we make another person responsible for defining our worth, we will try to control how that person feels about us. This creates many problems in relationships because it means we are trying to get love rather than share it. Only when we accept the responsibility of defining our own worth and learn to love ourselves will we have love to share with others.

When you make decisions for yourself that are healthy and based on your interests, needs, and feelings, you are demonstrating self-love. But when you make decisions against your interests, needs, and how you want to feel, it harms you and moves in a direction of unpleasant emotions or unfulfillment. And if you chose against your needs, you can't expect to have a life where your emotional intelligence invites safe, loving people into your life.

Practicing self-love starts with paying attention to how you feel. Pay attention to the decisions you make for yourself, the goals you set for yourself, and most importantly how you treat yourself every single day. Do the people around you inspire you? Who do you let into your life?

We often think about self-love in the form of having our nails done or buying a new outfit or new shoes. These are things outside of you that can give you instant gratification and the feeling of looking good. But if these things could give you real happiness, you wouldn't be reading this book. I am sure you have done all of these, but inner peace was nowhere to be found. Real self-love is the true essence of who you are. You believe in your dreams, and you are not afraid to stand up for yourself despite knowing that other people might not accept you. Real self-love means knowing what you deserve and that your self-worth can't be taken away.

Self-love takes practice. There are many forms of self-love, but the true essence of it is that you have a sense of being enough no matter what gets done in a day, what other people think of you, and how much they appreciate you.

Don't think for a second that loving yourself is self-centered or selfish. It is self-nurturing, self-expansive, interconnected, and conscious.

Many of us think that we should be complete to deserve something particular or perhaps to deserve anything. If you think this way, you will attract people in your life whose love depends on how you perform.

If you understand and resonate with a sense of acceptance and wholesomeness, you can accept everything about yourself—the flaws, the things you are still working on, and things that you haven't figured out yet but that you acknowledge. If you still feel that you deserve to love and be loved, you can change your life for the better.

Self-love is a choice from one moment to the next. It involves doing the work from the inside. It involves honoring your voice, feeling worthy enough no matter what, and going after your dreams and goals.

I'm pretty sure that if you are struggling with dieting, emotional eating, and body image insecurity, you don't have the necessarily skills yet to honor your voice or feel worthy enough to go after what makes you truly happy. If you were able to satisfy your emotional needs without food or working for the perfect body, you would have enough self-care tools in your pocket.

Don't hold back because of fear of what happened in the past. If you live in fear, you will never get to meet the real you. Don't hate where you are right now. Be grateful that you are seeking. If you are afraid of showing up in your life because you might lose something or somebody, ask yourself the following questions:

If I want to show up in my life with my real self and I disappoint people in the meantime, what does that mean?

Do they want the best for me?

Could they be getting something out of me not being myself?

Does that mean if I lose people because they don't like the new me, than should I really be around those people?

Is it worth more to love myself first, be who I really am, and have people who love me for that, or to pretend to be somebody else so that I can make people around me happy?

One thing is for sure. You'll take what is given to you based on the value you place on yourself. When you practice self-love, you will only settle for what you worthy of. Therefore, stand up for yourself when you need to. Stop people pleasing, and say no or yes based on how you feel. Build boundaries if you need to, and don't be afraid to ask for what you want. Instead of attacking people for how they treat you, let them know how their actions make you feel. Respect yourself for what you are going through. In society, we think there is no place for vulnerability, but there is. The only way to live a real life is to show up with your emotions. Self-love involves honoring the journey you have been on and seeing the gift. If you don't do that—regardless of how painful or difficult the situation you went through was—it will hold you back.

I was the victim of weight stigmas for two decades. I couldn't see the gift in my struggle with diets or body hate and instead just wanted to numb myself with food whenever I could. Being on my knees, looking for answers, was quite a journey. Only when I was willing to look behind the curtain at the root cause of my struggles was I able to heal and peace of mind. It didn't come by losing weight but by understanding the force driving my struggles.

The more you can tap into the feelings that connect you to your true self and dig deep, the more you will unleash the gift they offer you. Don't hold back. Every answer is inside of you. Self-love will help you get to the core of who you are. And when you have the courage to look into your dreams and desires and show up in your life, your physical appearance will change naturally rather than being a forced change. You don't want to live a life where you are merely surviving or that you sleepwalk through. You want a life where you can thrive in the essence of who you are.

Self-love is an action—you have to do something to demonstrate it. However, self-love is an act of being, not doing. Check in with yourself daily; honor your voice and whatever feelings come to you during the day. Make a mental note or write it down to acknowledge your feelings. Your voice matters. Tuning in to yourself a couple times a day can make you become aware of how you feel about the people around you and the things happening to you; you can choose to react and be true to yourself. Instead of only asking how you will make another person feel if you do this or that, ask yourself how you feel about what the other person said or did to you.

Regardless of why you developed poor emotional health and how you lack the skills to for mental and emotional stability no matter what happens outside of you, you can still cultivate them now. Instead of waiting for outside validation and reassurance that you are valuable, loveable, and worthy, you can work your way to feeling this way internally. When you are centered enough to have a sense of self-worth and self-love, your inside world will match your outside world. Sooner or later, all areas of your life, including the struggle with weight and your body, will naturally fall into place, and you will find peace with food and happiness with your body.

The Effects of Criticism

Alan Cohen once said, "I give myself the kindness and forgiveness I would show others."

The diet industry teaches you to spend money on their products to lose weight faster. Messages from ads, billboards, and the media in general want you to believe that the thinner you are, the happier you will be. You may feel a lot of frustration when you are not able to achieve or maintain your goal easily or at all. And then you do what was modeled for you: using self-criticism and negative self-talk toward yourself.

The root cause of the unhappiness underneath your weight struggle and compulsive eating is partly from the negative self-talk under every nasty comment you make about yourself. This negativity pushes you to do things with less flexibility to get the results you want. You might get short-term results, but it never really feels good, and it is hard for you to keep up.

Willpower and self-criticism are like best buddies. Up until now, you have likely used self-criticism to achieve your goals. How is that working out for you so far? When I mention self-criticism, I am referring to the voice inside you that comes up of its own accord. It often says things like, "I am not good enough," "I am worthless," or "I can't beat this."

We grow up believing that with a fair amount of self-criticism, we can push ourselves to be our best and feel good. We think it motivates us to become a fabulous achiever and that it doesn't really matter whether we are joyful in the process. Among women who have body image insecurity, self-loathing is a common practice. Critiquing one's appearance, focusing on imperfections and shortcomings, is in fact quite uncommon. This way of living can make it feel like there is an enemy living inside of you. Most of us grew up with self-criticism. We believe it's normal. I don't think I have met anyone in my entire life who naturally loves or shows kindness to themselves when they mess up.

When we use self-criticism, the amygdala—the oldest part of the brain—quickly detects threats in the environment, and the fight-or-flight response is triggered. The amygdala sends signals that increase blood pressure, adrenaline, and hormone cortisol, mobilizing the strength and energy needed to confront or avoid the perceived threat. This system evolved to deal with physical attacks, but it is activated just as readily by emotional attacks from others ourselves. So, when you are beating yourself up, you are activating all of these stress signals.

All of our emotional responses are related to a survival instinct. We get angry so that we can defend ourselves; we get sad so that we can elicit social support from others. The trick is learning how to start a relationship with ourselves so that our natural compassion toward others can be turned toward ourselves. It is a very interesting kind of dilemma, because we are the one who is suffering, and we also have to find a part of ourselves that can witness the suffering and have a relationship with that aspect of our person. Being critical with ourselves is a hardwired trait, so it is not something we are able to get rid of, but you can make it stop being in charge. Self-criticism toward the body often shows up as the thought that you want to disown it or get rid of it. It can feel like a sense of self-rejection or disconnection. Interestingly enough, Western culture places great emphasis on being kind to our friends, family, and neighbors, who are struggling. Not so when it comes to ourselves. When we make mistakes or fail in some way, we're more likely to hit ourselves over the head with something than comfort ourselves. It is time to start treating yourself as you would treat someone very close to your heart.

Even though you have been struggling with your weight for a long time, going on and off diets, you might not want to hear about working on your body image. But how has dieting and hating your body worked out so far?

If judgment and criticism have worked, then you each be in a loving relationship with yourself. If you are constantly checked out of your body and using all your mental energy for self-hate and pushing yourself to diet or lose weight, you cannot have a loving and nurturing relationship with yourself, which would give you what you are looking for. If judging, criticizing, and not approving of your body worked, you would be at your ideal body weight and have peace with your body. However, there are so many of us living in own fear, judgment, and criticism, whether we have body image insecurities or not. The truth is that when we live in a critical space, we close the door to having a sense of inner peace and happiness, no matter how many external things we are able to acquire. What do you want more: peace of mind or an ongoing struggle with food?

"You and your body are on the same side," said Brooke Castillo.

This quote emphasizes that your body is not your enemy; therefore, your life shouldn't be a battle between you and your body. The moment you realize that your only job in your weight struggle is to learn how to communicate better with your body and experience your feelings instead of eating them you are heading toward self-awareness.

I'm sure your first reaction to accepting your body is that if do so right now, while it doesn't look the way you prefer, you will never be able to change it. But this is not true.

Think about a relationship in your life where you feel love toward a person although the relationship is not perfect. I invite you to think the same way about your body and yourself. Since perfection doesn't exist in real life, you get to choose if your relationship with yourself will be compassionate and understanding or full of criticism and judgment. The latter ends up being a dysfunctional relationship, and it might break down and leave you completely disconnected. A relationship that is accepting, nurturing, loving, open, and beautiful is not perfect, but it is peaceful.

Since criticism, self-judgment, and restrictions have been giving you bumpy roads of self-loathing, you might want to enjoy journey of body acceptance from a different perspective. Therefore, if you can create space for self-love to enter and have the mental energy to feel compassionate, understanding, and tuned in to your body, you can transform your mind and body so that it feels good. Self-acceptance has to come before any transformation or self-improvement.

We spend so much time on wanting other people to like us; we know them better than we know ourselves. We study them, we hang out with them, and we admire their values and want to have the same ones. However, when you compare yourself to others instead of comparing your actions to your own dreams, you run the risk of minimizing yourself. Yet, we are essentially programed to compare ourselves to others. There is nothing wrong with that if we only identify things we admire in others and then look inside ourselves for our unique values. We might have the same traits we see in others without being able to recognize them because we expect them to appear in exactly the same form we see in others. If you can't go to the mirror and say, "Wow, I love you," and hug yourself, be present with yourself, and tell yourself you are an amazing person, then why would you expect the world to treat you that way? It starts within you.

Happiness is a state of mind, not a particular body size or shape. You are not broken; you don't have to be fixed. You only have to remember who you are without all the expectations you put on yourself or picked up from your environment.

When girls and women learn to stop looking at their imperfect bodies as flawed and start seeing value in what they feel connected to—if they can remember who they actually are—they become happier and no longer need food to numb out their tension and misery. Their bodies then release excess weight and no longer suffer from permanent resistance to weight loss and compulsive eating behaviors.

Self-criticism feels like having someone push you or bite you from behind to keep going, isn't it? In contrast, self-compassion is more like a string on the heart that pulls forward with clarity, self-love, and inner wisdom.

Christopher Germer said, "A moment of self-compassion can change your entire day. A string of such moments can change the course of your life."

When you can be kind, compassionate, respectful, and loving toward yourself, it is a completely different perspective than seeing yourself critically. Real transformation happens when you love yourself as much as you love others.

What Is Body Acceptance, and Why Do You Need It?

You need to recognize that your feelings of not being good enough or worthy enough are inside of you. These are the beliefs you pick up along the way. Therefore, wanting to prove your worth when you are around people is most likely a projection of internal struggle. Feeling valued and worthy completely starts on the inside. Similarly, happiness is in not outside of you. It is found when you can accept things as they are.

Considering what really lies behind your body image insecurity, it's easier to understand how accepting and loving your body as it is can help you reach permanent weight loss. By accepting and loving your body as it is, things start to transform without so much pushing.

An ongoing weight struggle is actually a deep internal issue that manifests in your weight. If you are reading this book, it's probably been years if not decades since you started focusing on fighting fat with nutrition and exercise. And you don't see the results because you are focusing on something that can't give long-term ones.

The excess weight is the manifestation of fear, uncertainty and living in scarcity mind-set. When you live this way, you will always need protection. When you feel scared, insecure and not good enough, your choice of protection will be food, hence the weight issues. We feel ashamed or guilty about the fact that we eat but we are not going anywhere with our real issues, since we are looking for it in the wrong places. And since we are not finding the solution for our weight battle, we are more scared than ever before.

When you approach your weight struggle from love and understanding instead of fear, restriction, and willpower, you can understand that love doesn't require perfection. It means you understand that while you are aiming for a better body, a car, a job, or a spouse, you get to enjoy the ride. And by the time you arrive, you will always have a different goal. This is the way things are.

And while there will be bumps on the road, you can take them as gifts instead of failures. In fact, when you look at your weight struggle from a place of love and acceptance, you truly understand that, even if you are not where you want to be, you are in the place you are now because there is a beautiful lesson for you to learn.

Perfectionism is impossible to satisfy. You can never really become happy and peaceful from the inside until you are appreciative and grateful for what you have right now. Seeing the value of accepting what you don't have is the first step to go where you want to be. As soon as you learn the lesson, you can move forward and welcome a new one. They never stop; new lessons will come into your life for as long as you are breathing.

Reasons to Accept Your Body

Body acceptance lessen the power food has over you. Aiming for the perfect body is possible, but actually getting it is not. Once you reach your goal, you will immediately want to change your body again. It is human nature to never stop aiming for something we think is better. You are using so much mental energy to think about food—the dos and don'ts—that you don't realize that the craziness around food originates from having body image insecurities, the driving force for food issues. The way to get a break from being crazy around food is to let go of control over your body. If you want to be free from food controlling your mind and body, you have to let go of your insecurity about body image.

One of the reasons that food has such an impact on your life is because you want to control your body. The moment you stop wanting to control your body, food becomes secondary. Isn't that amazing?

As long as you worry about your weight, you will always want to control food. This pushes you into the diet-binge cycle because of the restriction aspect. Body acceptance is therefore the key to overcoming weight struggles.

You are always going to have food issues unless you accept your body. Until you stop being afraid of gaining weight or getting off your diet, you will always criticize your eating choices. Additionally, you are always going to have issues with body image, body shame, fat shame, and weight management until you accept your body. But soon as you accept your body, food loses its power over you. And then you can finally have a normal life around food.

When you are in a do-or-die mood, hopeless and desperate to lose weight, it keeps you from looking at food without being afraid. Diet mentality and shame around food will be part of your life until you stop worrying about your body.

They feed on each other. The only reason you diet is because you were told that it is your only option to get control over your body. Food wouldn't be an issue in your life if there were another way to control your body. Although it seems that food is the primary issue, it isn't. Think about why you want to control your body so badly. Food is just a means. What's the underlying cause?

You Could Have a Lean Body and Still Hate It

To get to your ideal body weight, you essentially have the following two options:

Plan A:

You can pursue chronic dieting and exercising, which is usually done by willpower in the form of forcing, restricting, or avoiding certain foods. When you get to your ideal body weight or size, you look how you are supposed to, but there is still pain inside of you. If you lose weight by hating your body, you will still hate your body when you get to your ideal weight. This is how the cycle starts. You lose it and gain it back all the time. If this is not you, you must know someone who lost weight, and you thought she was really happy, but she wasn't. She still hated her body because she couldn't accept herself in the first place. When you try to solve an internal problem externally with diet and exercise, because your mind-set doesn't change, your look might be different, but you still feel the same inside. At some point, you will eat and do the things again that make you gain weight in the first place.

Plan B:

The other approach is to accept where you are right now and see the gift in your struggle. When you can do that, you will be able to connect with your inner wisdom for what you truly need to take care of your weight. When you can respect your issues and the struggle that manifests in chronic excess weight, your journey to your ideal body weight will be the reverse of the first option. It's not based on fear but of acceptance. Honoring and listening to what comes up in the form of emotions and feelings will create peace with food and with yourself.

Therefore, as mentioned previously, your problem is actually a gift. After many years of dieting and weight struggles, a lot of people give up and stop working on themselves. What if I told you to love your problems, and the solution will appear? Honor the work you need to do. You have struggles for a reason. Whether you like it or not, there is something to improve. When eating is triggered by the diet-binge cycle or by emotions you can't handle, it is the result of you being disconnected from your body and from who you really are. The reason you have been struggling with chronic weight fluctuations is that by focusing on the excess weight and diet, you ignore the root cause of your issue: your scarcity mind-set and negative thoughts.

Do the inner work instead of hating your body. Feel your feelings, listen to the guidance they give you, and act accordingly. Your success will be based on how much work you have done on yourself from the inside out. When we work on ourselves first and remember what our true desires are, it is amazing how the weight disappears. When you recognize all the limiting beliefs you have and all the noise from living in modern society, and when you accept who you truly are and act accordingly, you are demonstrating self-love and self-acceptance. When you open up to listen, to communicate, and most importantly to connect with yourself with love instead of fear, you will no longer choose food as a drug when things get rough. By following your true desire, you will do what's necessary, even if what lies beneath your struggle with weight is scary.

Focus on Positive Body Image

Our culture doesn't really support everyone having different body shapes and sizes. If you look at the media, it says we should all be one size and height. The taller and thinner you are, the better, right? Human diversity is portrayed as a bad thing. Instead of following the impossible, it's better to embrace what you have. Don't measure your worth based on expectations. Look into the relationships in your life where inner beauty is more important than looking a certain way. Instead of deprivation or emotional eating, practice letting go of negative commentary, and do your best with what you have instead of mourning what you don't have. Don't fall for the notion that happiness comes in one size. You can have it all. You just need to believe in it. Remember, you have the fat talk with yourself over and over again as a byproduct of living in modern society. You are vastly influenced by the expectations of this century, this decade, and this year. But your body doesn't make you who you are as a person, even if the media says it does. Now that you are aware of the false expectations regarding how your body is supposed to look so you are good enough or happy enough, understand that you are just as worthy as anybody else, regardless of how you look.

In order to stimulate the economy, we are constantly sold to by companies. They create internal senses of inadequacy in us. Advertisers don't really tell you how a product makes your life better. They tell you how a product makes you better. And if you believe this false message, your emotional well-being and self-image is at stake. When you can really understand this is happening, you will naturally respect yourself and act from that place in every areas of your life. If you are seeking freedom from negative body image, you must remain aware of your thoughts and feelings when you are taking messages from your environment and interacting with the world.

You need to approach the way you look at yourself from a different perspective. When you find yourself as important as your friends, family, and loved ones are, you will not take things out on your body. Losing yourself is not worth to any relationship is not worth it; at the end, it doesn't feel good for you.

Our society focuses so much on physical appearance and tells us that our body doesn't belong to us. The culture conditions us on how we are supposed to look, feel, and behave. The biggest impact you can make on your own happiness is taking back your power by knowing that your body, spirit, and mind are your domain. Your beauty, worth, and value aren't measured by the shape of your body or by your weight. If you think they are, you will attract only people who are hard on themselves when it comes to measuring up to cultural standards regarding body weight and shape. You should not be a slave of someone else's insecurities, as they will project their issues onto you.

Mothers have the opportunity to teach their daughters how they to feel about their bodies. If a mother controls her child's body and what she wears or tells her how she is supposed to look, then when the daughter goes out into the world, she will let society tell her how to look. Bringing our style into the world should be for more than just vanity or validation from others. I got caught up in the weight and body image struggle that millions of women and girls get wrapped up in every day. When we learn to accept ourselves, we automatically make other people learn to accept us. To me, beauty is about being comfortable in my own skin. It's about knowing and accepting who I am.

Look closely at how you self-sabotage yourself. Do you stay in relationships of any kind that are emotionally damaging to you? Do you pick friends or partners based on the level of love you think you deserve? If you feel unworthy in any area of life, your relationships could reflect the same. Do you hang out with girls who desperately want to fix their body?

Having connections with people who are emotionally damaging or destructive or allowing them to stay in your life is a mirror to the pain inside of your own mind. They reflect the bad feelings you have about yourself.

I understand that living in modern society puts tremendous pressure on you to be thin and beautiful. You try to meet expectations because you want to feel connected and accepted. I understand that. But if you don't clean up your self-talk and come from a place of loving yourself instead of tolerating the judging voice in your head, you will never be happy, even if you lose weight. You will have to overcome the fear of what people will think if you gain weight.

A positive body image can feel weird at first, and it is easy to judge it. But if you are able to recognize what triggers your negative body image and accept the fact that you can't be all of those things that society puts on you, you will appreciate yourself more. This is true not only because you understand the ridiculousness of those expectations but also because you will understand that even if you can get leaner, it doesn't necessary make you happy.

You will be treated with more love because you love yourself more, and you will not allow anyone to treat you otherwise. The more you can accept what's good in you because you want to be yourself, you will attract people who accept you and like you just the way you are, and this leads to happiness. But you have to stick with what you want and how you feel instead of doing, feeling or looking how other people require. You are already good enough, and when you can truly embrace it, others will as well.

If you strive to like your body, it's like living in a space of not liking it. When you are instead able to feel and visualize that you already have the body that you are aiming for, you will naturally be driven to do less damaging things to your body because you embrace it.

What Does Real Happiness Have to Do with Body Acceptance?

As I said earlier, I think you are beautiful the way you are, but if losing weight is something that you want to pursue to have a healthy looking body, that's okay. But if you want to lose weight in the hope of solving your problems with insecurities, doubts, fear, and loneliness and to have lasting satisfaction, you have the wrong goal in mind. If you believe by reaching your goal in terms of losing weight that you are going to directly head toward happiness, success, and peace of mind from food and body image issues, I hate to be the buzzkill, but it won't happen.

Chronic dieters, binge eaters, overeaters, and others whose weight fluctuates most of the time are not any happier after they lose the weight. The external validation can't give them what they are truly looking for in losing weight. It feels good to get a gold star or a look of acknowledgment from someone you respect. However, this kind of validation is fleeting because it's not yours to own. If you don't do inner work to own your value, this goodness will slip away.

When you get validation from others, it is about what they think of you. Of course it feels good, but if you think you look good only when you get confirmation from others, what happens when they stop complimenting you? If you are constantly depending on others to make you feel good about yourself, it is like waiting on somebody for your happiness.

Aiming for a better body because of expectations form others is an external pursuit that will never fulfill your soul. We are internal beings first.

Until you can be happy with yourself as you are right now, you will never be happy with any external changes. The environment makes you believe that when you get validation from others or if you get certain things in your life, you will be happy. But true happiness can only be experienced if you are happy on the inside first.

Lean Toward Inner Peace to Be Happy

The less you think that your ultimate happiness can only be found in a perfect body, the more you are headed toward a happiness that creates inner peace.

Continue on your journey and be committed, curious, and resilient in spirit. As recommended previously, be compassionate with yourself and treat yourself with love. Look at your failures as learning lessons. You are imperfectly perfect. Your challenges are not life sentences. Behavior can be changed with time.

Continue regardless of setbacks, and you will be on your way to developing new skills and setting yourself up for long-term success. Your body is like a chemistry lab" an ever-changing miracle. You change along with your circumstances from one second to another, and it will be like this for the rest of your life. Everything outside of you can change over time, but if you allow it to develop, the only thing that won't change is the acceptance and internal love you can feel toward yourself regardless of your circumstances.

Things outside of you can give you enjoyment and pleasure; there is no doubt about it. Opinions from others can be flattering. But all the external things are by definition an outside world. And if you live by those rules, your life can feel like a victory or like misery.

If you can truly embrace the fact that you are worthy, lovable, and valuable in every way, you can find true happiness.

Many people I've met who have it all are far from being happy. They are always moving on the next thing, and they let their circumstances define who they are and what their worth is. It is a never-ending battle. But you can't buy internal nourishment. As the saying goes, you can't buy happiness. All the things outside of you are just temporary fixes. You are happy when you get them, but the excitement goes away, and want to get the next thing.

Having the goal for a better body and being passionate about it is important if that's what makes you excited. External pursuits are not bad things. But if you feel that it is your only source of peace and success, you are chasing something that you can never catch.

Don't miss out on today; tomorrow will never come. If you love yourself now, the decisions you are making today can only lead to a life of sustainable happiness. For a long time, there were a lot of reasons I didn't love myself, and this was something I had to work on every day. I didn't really think I was good enough to do the things I wanted to do, and it was a battle for worthiness all along.

Now that I have a different view on life, I ask myself the following questions almost every day:

- Do I do this to justify my existence here?
- Do I have the mind-set that once I reach this goal, I will be more worthy of love and better able to love and accept myself?

If my answer is yes, I know I need to do some inner work. All of my success can be taken away, but if I stand on a solid belief that I am worthy of love and belonging no matter what, I can always remake anything external. Let go of resistance today and love yourself right now. I promise that it will bring everlasting satisfaction and success. The only way to build a strong foundation of being yourself" is to do what feels right inside of you. When you are able to honor your emotions and feelings, you respect who you are. And once you make better choices because you are thinking and operating out of respect, that's when permanent body transformation happens.

Be Willing to Change

If you have been struggling for a while with compulsive eating, on-and-off dieting, or resistance to permanent weight loss, I am sure you use some tools to try to make permanent change.

How is it working for you so far?

I am asking because I know for sure that even if we want transformation, the desire is not enough. The willingness needs to be filled with a feeling of hitting the bottom hard enough to wake up ready to do this. If you are not ready to have a shift in your perception, it is going to be difficult to get lasting results.

When you are committed to your own point of view, even if you say you want change, you are not really ready to let go. I believe willingness is a bit of magic. But again, unless you hit bottom, a shift in your perception will barely occur. However, the fact that you are reading this book is a sign that a shift in perception might be on the way.

The willingness to let go what doesn't work and try something new sounds easy. We would like it to come naturally, but that doesn't necessarily happen. And there is a reason for this. The kind of shift I am talking about doesn't involve an instant outside force giving you the tools. It comes from within.

The catalyst that made me want to see things differently came from all the years that I tried so hard to control my body. Remember, at the beginning of the book, I mentioned that I found it too difficult to stay at my ideal body weight, and I wasn't even happy when I arrived. I had the same unworthiness crisis and negative self-talk from time to time, even though my body had changed.

Stefanie Nielsen, writes in her book *You Can Overcome Binge Eating*, "If your desire, your reason why, is not big enough, you will struggle. Or if you have more reasons to fail than to succeed … you will fail.

If it is still more comfortable for you to stay in the place you are, then you will."

We turn to food because we don't understand what's missing in our life, or we don't have the capability to move past our emotions and feelings. We lack adult self-care.

The shift in perception we need can come in many ways. For example, it can happen when you are given some guidance that hits home or you are fed up with doing the same thing again without seeing results, or you might get inspired to be a role model to others. The reasons we want to change are endless. But there has to be a trigger point that changes your whole perspective on your ongoing problem. The desire has to come from within, and I believe it needs to be connected to something bigger than you.

Don't fall for the old way of thinking, meaning you just ignore your issues that that trigger emotional eating, forcing yourself to look good by rigid diet and exercise plans, and then waiting to suddenly become self-confident and self-accepting.

Making your body weight and shape responsible for your happiness is a dead end. As mentioned previously, living from a place of appreciation for wherever you are on your journey—whatever you experienced so far—and focusing on learning about yourself will give you the true happiness.

Finding what brings you peace or joy is the real task. Remember, your struggle with weight is there to teach you a lesson like all struggles are. Allow yourself to know what brings you back to emotional balance. Experience joy by daring to be who you are and not pretending to be someone you are supposed to be.

Act According to How You Want to Feel

One of the hardest things to do in any kind of transformations is getting what we want without forcing it or relying on willpower. As human beings, by default, we are a bunch of fearful folks who want to fit into society, and our inner critic makes sure we stick with things that feel familiar.

My favorite quote from Wayne Dyer is, "I will attract into my life what I am, not what I want." It has been life changing in my transformation and I am sure it has been to many others. It took me a long time to truly understand what he meant.

You don't attract things into your life based on what you want, whether it is to get a thin body, to stop eating emotionally, or to stop hating your body because so much of wanting is living in the space of what you don't have. You don't become thin by wanting to become thin. By constantly telling yourself how fat you are and that you need to lose weight in order to be someone important, it is like living in a space of not being someone.

It doesn't matter what you wish you were or what your goal is if you can't immerse yourself in the idea of how sexy and thin you already are in your mind, even if physically you aren't there yet.

What you did in the past led you to where you are right now. The way you thought about life and the way you ate was the result of your beliefs, thoughts, feelings, emotions, and actions. Did you use willpower to gain weight? My guess is that you didn't. You lived with a mind-set that resulted in weight gain. The same is true for permanent weight loss. When you get to a point where your mind-set—beliefs, thoughts, feelings, and emotions—is what makes you lose the weight, you will naturally manifest the body you want. But for this to happen, you need to live in a space of picturing yourself as thin. You are the creator of your mental pictures. It is like creating a movie, and you are the lead actor.

Being able to act as if you are thin or feminine is a great stepping-stone in your process of transformation. When you can consciously visualize vivid details because you believe you truly deserve and get what you want, you will move forward, drawing actions and results into your life not because you want them, but because you are those things already without physically having them yet. When you imagine how you want your body to appear, it helps to your cells to record this state of being in their memory, and then you are own your way to being who you already are. Always give your attention to what you want instead of what you don't want. This is how you can get closer to having anything you want in life.

When you understand this, you will see how the people around you are at certain places in life that demonstrate the beliefs about they have about themselves. It is like common sense.

Another turning point occurs when we work on gradually increasing our awareness of what we believe about our worth and knowing how what we think we deserve.

Your failure to stop eating compulsively or dieting over the past several years might not have been because of your willpower or lack thereof. I am sure you can see the connection by now indicating why you can be successful in other areas of your life but here. With all the knowledge and success you acquired along the way, perhaps you wondered why you were not able to do what you were supposed to do.

You believed that you were focusing on the problem (dieting, emotional eating, and body shame), but they are only the effect of the real issue underneath. Now you know you've been focusing on the effect all along.

Awareness is the first step, and you are already there. Understanding who you are in your thoughts and beliefs that you make decisions on is a big part of understanding everything you do and why you do it. In order to let go of the pain, shame, fear, or worry that creates your extra weight as well as the tendency to eat compulsively or experience body shame, you must understand what shapes these issues in the first place. You must change from within before the outside changes. Instead of thinking you need to fix yourself, I invite you to think differently about what's ahead of you on the journey of transformation. Your job is to pay attention, to be curious, and to show up for you feelings. Look behind the beliefs shaping your life. More specifically, look behind everything you believe about why dieting will save you, why binging is not what you really want to do, even though it feels good for a while, and why focusing on body image insecurity gets in the way of seeing what really bothers you. When you can believe that you have the answers to your problems within you, you will no longer choose food to shut your feelings down. You will no longer want to focus on diets to save you from insecurity and shame. When you no longer believe something is inherently wrong with you, you will take on new beliefs that shape a life you want to live. When your beliefs are different from the reality you want to live, and you want to be someone you are not, you will eventually understand that everything you want is in you. Wanting it is what makes it feel like you don't have it.

Questioning your core beliefs can be intimidating at first. Who are you without your beliefs? How would you decide right before binging if somehow, suddenly your beliefs were different from the thing that triggered binging in the first place? The solution lies in observing your beliefs based on the stories you tell yourself and what you sense—how you feel—in your body. Emotional vulnerability is crucial to seeing who you really are. Instead of running away, you are standing in the face of your feelings and their gifts, even if it feels weird and unusual to stay with your feelings.

Part V
How to Transform Your Body through Nutrition

Knowing that I am a nutritionist, you would probably think that I was mostly going to talk about the health benefits of foods and what foods you need to eat to lose or manage your weight. However, although I worked with nutrition for a while to lose weight or manage my clients' weight, after many years of struggles, I needed to look for answers somewhere else. We all know how to lose weight; this is not the problem anymore. What troubles most people is how to keep it off.

Even professionals like doctors, dietitians, and nutritionists typically think that the main reasons for weight gain or unsuccessful weight management is slow metabolism, overeating, or bad genetics. But none of these conditions actually causes our issues. As mentioned previously, your problem is actually an external reflection of deep internal issues. For example, the effect of weight fluctuations is a signal of emotional weight you carry in your body. I don't believe that people have an obsession with food and engage in compulsive eating because they have 'genes predisposing them to sugar addiction or because drug-like foods exist that are addictive because the food tastes so good.

I think people become addicted or obsessed with food and eat compulsively (whether via the diet-binge cycle or emotional eating) because how they feel about themselves is highly influenced by the relationship they have with food. Because people who have weight issues let their food choice dictate how they feel about themselves, they also let their weight dictate how much they love themselves. Food has enormous power over us; whether we restrict our food intake or overeat, we think our success in relation to food can be a great baseline for our future success in life. As silly as it sounds, this is the truth. In our culture, being skinny is the gateway to success at work, in relationships, and generally in life. Based on cultural expectations, happiness depends on your body;

it will make or break whether you are respected, loved, or accepted in all areas of your life. Hopefully, just be reading this make you aware of how ridiculous it is to base your body on your success, no matter what society tells you. When you can change your relationship with your body, you have a shot at changing your relationship with food. Until then, food will always have power over you.

I am not going to give you a diet plan to stick with. The best diets are the ones where you can turn a nutrition plan into a lifestyle that allows you to lose fat or manage your weight because you have a healthy relationship with food. The effects of food are not just physical; they are also mental and emotional.

My intention with this chapter isn't to give you information about healthy eating. Chronic dieters could become nutrition experts. But they might not know the following things about weight management and nutrition:

- What normal eating is and how you can change your relationship to food
- How to regulate blood sugar after meals without being hungry or having cravings
- How calories in food impact fat-burning and fat-storing hormones

Brooke Castillo said, "No diet can substitute for the wisdom of your body."

Most of the times when we want to fix our body, we look for a diet or nutrition plan to fix us, and then we rigidly follow the food rules it provides. When you do that, you can easily get disconnected from your own body and ignore its signal for whether you are hungry or not. Part of my plan is to encourage you to tune in to how your body feels. I invite you to get to know how it feels when it communicates via hunger and fullness. If you are a chronic dieter, it will take some practice and willingness.

The Purpose of Eating

Food can be used for different experiences, most of which are in the following categories:

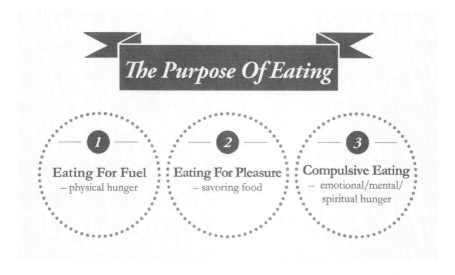

- **Eating for Fuel**—Eating out of physical hunger in order to nourish the body with the nutrients it needs to be able to function healthy and properly.
- **Joyful Eating for Pure Pleasure**—The outcome of this type of eating is that you feel good after eating. You don't think about it much other than feeling the pure joy of it.
- **Compulsive Eating**—An out-of-balance emotional state turns into emotional binging, including overeating, zoning out on food, and filling up on food to feel emotionally satiated. Although the food you eat comforts you, it leaves you feeling drained, sick, disappointed, ashamed, and guilty.

I am going to be brutally honest with you. Emotional eating is not something that will ever go away. You need to understand this, take a deep breath, and let it out. You can always have a moment or a split second in your life when your emotions will drive you to eat. It is a very human thing to do.

But the more you engage in different things than grabbing food when you feel the need to numb your feelings, the less frequent this instant craving will make you want to use food to dull the edge. When you get used to listening to your body, and you are aware of when emotional imbalances drive you to cope with food, you can catch it and choose a different path to handle your emotions; that is, you can choose not to eat compulsively anymore, ever. But it takes practice. And sometimes the practice includes eating emotionally when you feel like there is nothing else you can do. Don't beat yourself up.

Hunger versus Craving

It is important to start paying attention to your feelings of hunger. You will notice that much of what you've labeled hunger is actually something else. What you sense might be you feeling anxious, happy, sad, angry, uncertain, bored, or lonely. There is a huge difference between physical hunger and emotional craving. So how do you know the difference? Interestingly enough, a lot of times people don't see the connection between mood and food, and they think, "Oh, I am just hungry," and they eat. But eating has nothing to do with real hunger. How can you become aware of when you eat based on an out-of-balance emotional state?

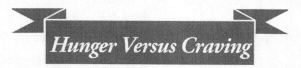

Hunger Versus Craving

The difference between hunger (physical) and cravings (emotional)

Physical hunger happens out of physical need. The hunger occurs because it has been a couple of hours since last time you ate. Your energy is getting low, blood sugar drops and you might even experience light-headedness. **Craving** can come with full stomach and it has to do with an emotional charge in you. Someone either did something, said something or you feel something and suddenly you want to eat.

Physical hunger is physically felt in your body in the gut and there is a need to fill the emptiness there. Your stomach has sensations. It rumbles first then later it growls. **Emotional craving** for food is felt in the heart or above the neck, in the head or in the mouth. A craving is more subconscious, under the radar and there is a need to fill the emptiness in your mind or in your heart.

Physical hunger is gradual and eating can wait. Physical hunger gives you steadily progressive clues about the feeling of hunger, it occurs gradually. **Craving** is different. One minute you are not even thinking about food but the next minute you are starving to death. You have a sudden urge to eat.

Physical hunger leaves you open to eat a variety of food. You might have certain options in mind but you are flexible. You are open to alternative choices. **Craving** goes for a specific food in mind. There is no alternative option. You mind exactly knows what it wants. It is specific.

When you eat out of **physical hunger**, it is easy to stop for you when you don't feel hungry anymore. **Emotional eating** doesn't let you stop when you are full; you are more likely to keep eating. It's like using food when certain emotions trigger feelings that are all over the place in you and you need to zone out on food. Although your stomach might be hurting from being overly full, somehow you feel peaceful again and then your appetite dissipates.

Physical hunger leaves you feeling good after eating. You feel you filled up a necessity in your eating, a biological need like breathing or sleeping. You consider it a necessary behavior. **Emotional eating** can leave you with bad feelings such as shame, guilt and regret. You feel like your self-worth is on the line. You feel bad about yourself.

When you are **physically hungry** and eat, you are present, calm and you consciously choose whether to eat everything on your plate or leave behind some of it. **Emotional eating** is absentminded eating. You don't really taste the food. You are on an automatic pilot. You are zoned out. The energy you bring around food is frenetic, controlled, fast, scared or mindless.

You might think based on what you read above that whenever you're not eating out of physical hunger, it is emotional eating. Luckily, this is not the case. Children and adults all eat emotionally and use food as a tranquilizer from time to time, and that's fine. Food is also for joy and pleasure. But for many people, food has power over them. They use and overuse food as a way of coping, and sooner or later, it becomes their habitual method for dealing with emotions.

Joyful Eating versus Filling Up on Food

Many emotional eaters say that eating makes them happy. In the moment of pursuing happiness, food is there to help. I get it. It is a habit of many girls and women.

But there is a difference between happiness and numbness. When you feel happy, you feel recharged, but when you are numb, that's only temporary relief from pain. It is just a matter of time before you feel it.

The problem is that the line between happiness and numbness has become blurred. Compulsive eating is not happiness.

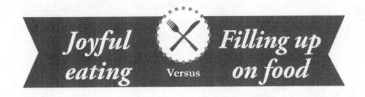

Joyful *eating*	*Filling up on food* *for self-shooting*
Being in a joyful relationship with food by eating for pleasure and cultural experience	Eating as a way of numbing is not happiness — it's temporary relief from pain
You feel happy and re-charged after eating	You eat to escape from your body
You eat for the love of food that feels good to you even after eating	You eat to zone out from your mind/thoughts
No bad feelings followed by about what you consumed	You eat to escape from your emotions

Eating as a cultural experience is wonderful. Enjoying any meal offers happiness, but emotional eating is not about that. It typically involves high sugar and high fat signals being sent to the brain, and feelings of guilt and shame follow.

Many times, my clients ask if a healthy nutrition plan means being away from sweets or desserts for good. This would be a total diet mentality, wherein restrictions can only lead to binges.

Food is very soothing because it changes our body chemistry and hormones and eventually adjusts how we feel. When you eat for nourishment and for the love of food, it is absolutely fine, and it gives you pleasure and joy. If you eat to comfort yourself in moderation to ward off a blue mood or to give yourself something as a reward on rare occasions, it is also fine. Food is meant for celebration and relief. People who have no issue with food eat emotionally sometimes. It's part of being human. But there is huge difference between making occasional mood fixes with food and doing it compulsively as your dominant coping mechanism to deal with different mood states.

If you eat desert, although that's not usually eating for fuel—for physical hunger—but rather for the joy of pleasure in the experience, it can enrich your life, and it is wonderful. It has nothing to do with covering up, hiding out, or controlling an emotion you don't want to feel. And it has nothing to do with binging, numbing, overeating, or the feelings of unworthiness that comes after that.

On the other hand, wolfing down an entire candy bar or an entire bag of chips when you are sad, happy, or about to have a sensitive discussion about something important has nothing to do with pleasure or joy. It is eating for comfort, to fill up the void inside of you. Your feeling of self-worth is most likely on the line as well. But while the food stuffs you to the point of being uncomfortable, there is still a hollow place for emotions. It's a void you can't seem to fill.

When you take a break to watch your favorite show, it is entertaining. You enjoy every moment of it, and when you are done, you feel reenergized and happy. But when you turn the TV on to zone out without actually being interested in what you are watching, and you don't gain much pleasure when you are done, it feels very different. You feel guilty and it indicates you're avoiding something in your life.

Whether you eat because you are physically hungry, because you want to indulge and enjoy food, or because you want to fill up the emptiness inside of you, food will always have an emotional effect. That's why it is used for so many reasons. When you eat to handle emotions, food pretty much feels like a weapon against the emotion lingering inside you.

The goal is to know the difference between eating for enjoyment and eating to block your emotions. As long as you are eating with inner freedom rather than driven by fear, you are good to go.

Most people eat to soothe their feelings occasionally. It is so common that we can all identify with the phrase "comfort eating." But if you put shame and self-hate around eating, that's not healthy or productive. How do you know when you have a healthy relationship with food?

The following are clues to check for during or after eating:

- You don't beat yourself up, and you don't feel bad about yourself for eating.
- You don't think your optional weight gain can be a roadblock to feeling worthy, accepting yourself, or feeling happy.
- You feel emotionally uplifted and don't have bad feelings regarding your sense of self.
- You might make a general note to yourself to eat healthier, but your baseline of self-worth, self-love, and self-acceptance is intact.

How to You Realize if You Eat Emotionally

First, you need to eliminate the diet mind-set so that you can get rid off the diet-binge cycle. When you remove the potential for binge eating because you are not on a diet, you immediately create an environment to override limiting or restricting diet lifestyles. You simply eat for the cultural experience, or you acknowledge that you are eating for emotional nourishment. You have to get rid of the diet mind-set first. If you don't get rid of this layer, you can confuse emotional eating with the diet-binge cycle, and these are two different things. One type of compulsive eating, the diet-binge cycle, occurs because of the restrictions; the other type of compulsive eating occurs as a reaction to an out-of-balance emotional state. If you have eliminated the diet mind-set and you are not physically hungry, you can decide why you are eating each time. When you eat for joy and pleasure, your self-worth is not on the line, and your moral character doesn't get damaged.

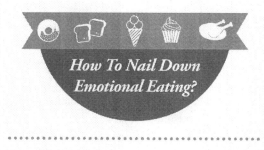

How To Nail Down Emotional Eating?

Compulsive eating can occur because of food restriction or out of balance emotional state.

Get rid of the diet mindset layer first.

Get off dieting in order to overcome the diet-binge cycle.

Diets don't resolve binge eating they feed on them.

Deprivation, restriction, pushing, shame and guilt around dieting is actually a straightjacket for binging or overeating.

If you are not on a diet, you can't push yourself to the binge cycle, out of deprivation.

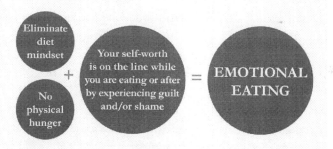

Your Nutrition Plan Is Normal Eating

The relationship you have with food is a perfect mirror for the relationship you have with yourself and with life.

Whether your goal is to lose weight (or fat) or to manage your weight, what you eat is an important factor. Before I go into nutrition, I want to be frank with you. I am not going to tell you how many times you are supposed to eat per day or how frequently. I am not going to give you a diet plan or tell you anything specific about whether you should eat grains, dairy, or legumes. These food groups are often called trigger foods by the diet industry, and people who have weight issues supposedly can't have them. I lived most of my life this way, and I never kept my weight.

However, I eat all of them now, and I am lean. I am not triggered by eating them anymore, so I have them regularly. It is a mind-set thing. You might get it now, or you might get it later. My hope is that you will get it eventually, and you can experience the freedom of eating these foods frequently without feeling guilty, ashamed, or bad.

I am suggesting that unless you have an allergic reaction or sensitivity to a certain kind food, don't avoid it just because some experts have said they make you gain weight What makes you gain weight is the fact that you can't have them; this triggers a sense of deprivation and rebellion in you, so the more you deny yourself the food, the more you want it. It is that simple. I wish someone had told me the same thing twenty years ago.

While working with clients and spending a couple of years working in health clubs, I had the opportunity to have long conversations with people who are so-called normal eaters. They eat grains, legumes, and starchy vegetables, and eating them regularly doesn't trigger these people to eat more.

No matter whether I interviewed a leaner or a bigger person— anyone who was not concerned about their weight and not on diets— they had a special relationship with the so-called trigger foods that I didn't understand for a long time. They told me that since they can have trigger foods anytime and are not afraid of the food, they don't want them all the time. They can leave trigger foods on their plate if they were physically satisfied.

I spent so much time with people who were afraid of food—friends and clients, not to mention myself—that I didn't understand immediately what these normal eaters meant. A bunch of people don't give a hoot about food shame. They are not sucked into the vortex of thinking they have to be a certain size to be good enough, so they actually eat when they are hungry and stop when they are full. They eat healthfully but not at the expense of avoiding high carbs just because it could make them gain weight or trigger certain reactions. Somehow these people manage their weight just fine because they don't eat compulsively for any of the reasons discussed earlier in this book.

Normal eating is very simple, but it is not necessarily easily. It requires having a clean state of mind, wherein you don't listen to the noises of the outside but only those of the inside. You feel when you are hungry rather than thinking you are hungry. You don't eat based on a clock but based on feelings of physical hunger. You don't change your eating patterns because of your lifestyle; instead, you support eating, a basic need, with your lifestyle.

Additionally, normal eating requires living in a space where you welcome your hunger and are not afraid of true hunger like years of chronic dieting taught you to do. Instead, you know you can trust your hunger regarding how much food your body needs, and you don't become a victim of your mind. When you were an infant and small child, you intuitively knew when you were hungry, and you stopped before you overate. I want you to do the same from now on.

The human body is designed to be able to balance calorie intake with signals of satiety and fullness. I am sure you have noticed you feel hungrier some days than others. Multiple things can influence your true physical hunger, including how active or stressed you are, where you are in your menstrual cycle, and so on. Everything we do, eat, think, or feel impacts hormones and neurotransmitters. Hormones and neurotransmitters communicate throughout your brain and body. They tell your lungs to breathe, your heart to beat, and your stomach to digest food and drink. They also affect your mood, weight, and concentration.

It is good to have routines in your life, including with your eating habits. For example, you can learn to understand how your body reacts to food and what signals your body gives when it reaches hunger.

I have already talked about the line between physical and emotional hunger in the previous chapter and how easily you may confuse the two. Any of the following symptoms may represent physical hunger for you:

- Empty stomach
- Headache
- Irritability
- Low energy or fatigue
- Shakiness
- Difficulty concentrating
- Stomach gurgling, growling, or making rumbling noises
- Feeling hunger pangs
- Weakness or lightheadedness
- Faintness
- Low blood sugar

The Basics of Normal Eating

Tuning in with your body is not necessarily a thought; it is a sensation in your body. Physical symptoms indicate true hunger. Hunger that starts in the mind is referred to as emotional hunger.

Therefore, tuning in with your body means actually feeling you are hungry and not thinking you are hungry. If it is hard for you to understand the difference between physical hunger and mental hunger, I recommend you ask yourself the following questions:

- Where do I feel physical or biological hunger in my body?
- Am I able to feel the hunger cues of my body?

Food journaling can help you tune in to your body, but some people can't stand it. If you choose to do it, it is important to take notes about how your body feels when it is hungry or full. It is not about tracking calories or the amount you eat. This takes practice, ladies, so do not judge yourself or beat yourself up.

The concept of normal eating helps you with fat loss and helps you manage your weight after you have reached your ideal body composition. Specifically, the idea is to eat when you feel physically hungry and to stop when you feel a stretching sensation in the stomach; this means you are about to become full. It is more a state of being than doing. In other words, this is not another rule to keep your mind occupied.

Doug J. Lisle, PhD, and Alan Goldhamer, DC, authors of *The Pleasure Tap* call the "stretch sensation" a satiety mechanism. Their book explains that because our brains are built to sense the caloric value of foods and the hormonal impact, when we've eaten enough, our hunger drive is designed to shut down naturally. This ability was built into your psychology, as it is in the natural biological heritage of all humans. The satiety mechanism depends upon two types of receptors in your mouths and stomachs. They are called "stretch receptors," which give your brain information about how "stretched out" your stomach is, and nutrient receptors, which will tell you the density of nutrients in the food you have eaten.

Being able to tune in to your body because you believe it can give you the signals when you had enough food is important for weight management. Trust your biological signals, as they were designed to make sure you had enough.

Interestingly enough, eating when you feel physically hungry and stopping when you feel the stretching sensation in the stomach doesn't work for most people who have weight management issues. After years of chronic dieting, they have hunger, craving, and blood sugar fluctuation issues most of the time, so they need to develop a sensible eating plan to deal with their hunger and cravings.

Normal eating disagrees with the mainstream idea that your eating frequency should be dictated by a standard formula, such as: "Eat four to six meals a day to lose fat," "eating is simple; just eat when you are hungry," "eat food, not too much—mostly plants," "just choose vegetables instead," or "breakfast is the most important meal of the day." These are misleading recommendations, and you wouldn't be reading this book if any of them had worked for you in the long run. The diet industry created generations of women who believe they need to force-feed themselves at certain times to see results.

Normal eating helps you to regulate your blood sugar. This is because eating meals that keep your blood sugar even will give you mental clarity, good moods, hormonal balance, and fat loss. Whether your goal is weight management or fat loss, regulating your blood sugar is crucial.

As a method, normal eating advocates getting to know your personal metabolism and adjusting your approach accordingly. Your eating frequency should be determined by your ability to take care of your hunger, your energy, and your cravings, not by an arbitrary rule that works for a hypothetical individual. Find an eating pattern that works best for you. The right one should keep you full, eliminate cravings, and keep your energy balanced.

Guidelines for Normal Eating

The more rules you create around food and your daily nutrition intake, the more food will control your life.

Notice Your Hunger Signals

Normal eaters tend to notice their hunger signals, and they respond to them. They don't ignore them or experience them in a fearful way.

Don't Comment on Your Moral Character Regarding What You Eat

Normal eaters seek out a variety of food to fulfill their hunger. They may still have certain internal beliefs about what they want or don't want to eat; it is not that these people don't have any no-no foods. But there is a huge difference between the way people on diets react to eating something that they are not supposed to and the way normal eaters do: The latter people don't comment on their moral character. Countless women and girls have certain foods they avoid in their daily nutrition (like going gluten free, no grains, no meat, etc.). If these food plans are backed up with an internal belief and inner freedom, that's very different than being driven by fear. They are not limiting those foods just for the sake of restricting themselves, which ultimately creates symptoms of deprivation. Very different emotions and feelings are attached to these two approaches. Can you see the difference?

Check in with Your Hunger Cues before Eating

Every time you think you are hungry, listen to your hunger cues and ask yourself the following questions:

- Am I really hungry?
- What are my physical symptoms of being hungry?

Listen to your physical hunger cues, and when your body says, "Feed me," it is okay to eat. What if you want to eat when you are not hungry? It might be when you are alone or at a social gathering, and food looks so good and readily available. Don't judge yourself. Be compassionate. Whether you choose to eat or not, try to understand what's going on in your life that makes you want to eat.

Implement Preemptive Eating

If you know you have a tendency to become shaky as a sign of low blood sugar by the time you sense physical hunger, implement snacking, mini meals, or preemptive eating.

Be Present with Food while You Eat

Be in the now when you eat. Get centered. This requires the ability to connect with yourself and not feel weird about it. Taking three long breaths in and out is a good start, or say a word that makes you feel calm before you begin your meal. The more absent-minded you are while you are eating, the more you will feel like you missed your meal when you are done. If you are thinking, doing, or feeling everything else except your food, you can easily overeat because you are not tuned in to your body's signals. For example, if you are overwhelmed with emotions while you eat, you might just keep going in an attempt to stuff down whatever you are thinking about. Don't be a vacuum eater. Taste the food and its texture as you eat. If you actually take the time to love and enjoy your food, it can be a source of pleasure in your life.

Stretch Sensation

Get familiar with the stretch sensation described previously, and notice when you feel its signals. If it feels difficult to stop eating, check in with your feelings and thoughts. Check your HEC to recognize how energized you feel from food. HEC is stands for hunger, energy and cravings level and it is used by Dr. Jade Teta, Integrative Physician, author of The Metabolic Effect Diet.

Forget about the Clean-Your-Plate Policy

Don't worry about leaving food on your plate when you are done. Cleaning your plate will do no good for your waistline, and it will not save children in Africa. Normal eaters leave food on the plate if they are not hungry, and they don't think about arbitrary definitions of appropriate portion size. They notice their hunger level and then stop because they are experience fullness in the stomach.

Awareness about Different Styles of Eating

Intuitive eating or mindfulness eating is the closest thing to normal eating: consuming food when you are hungry and stopping when satisfied—also called the hunger-and-fullness diet—but it can only became a successful eating style if you do it without the diet mentality.

In other words, normal eating only works if you truly are not creating new boundaries around food and eating based on biological signals, and you stop eating as soon as your mind detects fullness. It takes so much mental energy to pay attention to mindfulness eating that it might become just another rule for eating if you're not careful. It can easily become a minefield of judgment regarding your performance and attitude around food. However, don't look at mindfulness eating as another rule that sets off shame triggers if you somehow eat when you are not hungry. The same goes for the biofeedback tools, such as HEC. Checking in with your hunger signal, energy levels, and cravings is something to be aware of, but don't look at it as a rigid boundary.

Don't think for a second that if you missed checking in with these clues, you are bad. The only way to experience a natural attitude around food is recognizing the experience when you eat and are not thinking about what you are supposed to eat or do. With willpower-based diets, your mind rules what you are supposed to eat; with intuitive eating diets, your body rules what you are supposed to eat; and with emotional eating diets, your emotions rule your eating pattern. With normal eating, I am trying to teach you to never let any of these dieting thinking patterns tell you that you are bad.. Creating peace around food is your primary goal to create freedom from ongoing weight fluctuates.

What about rules like sit down while you eat, don't talk while you eat, don't read anything while you eat, and so forth? Without commenting on these rules one by one, I would like to invite you to think about something. The activities you do or don't do while eating is not the most important thing. The energy you bring to the table is the most important thing. If you feel like looking out your window and standing up while you eat, and this is how you connect with food, feel free to do it. No one, not even me, can tell you what makes you feel relaxed and connected to food while you are eating. The relaxed energy vibrations and feelings you create while you are eating are important, but how you reach them is unique. Overall, if you can eliminate guilt and shame around your eating habits, you will binge less, overeat less, and eventually your reactive eating patterns will go away. You will no longer manifest emotional eating in your life.

When you are miserable enough to stop choosing food as your source of soothing and comfort, you will start implementing everything you have learned here. You might be uncertain about sensing your emotions, and that's why you want food to distract you as a quick fix. You might still want to numb your feelings or zone out on food. That's okay. When you are ready, you will start practicing the self-care tools, because you are ready for the change.

Food Is Pleasure

The sensation and the quality of the food satisfy us, not the quantity of it. If you can truly be present when you eat, and if you can taste and enjoy your food without eating fast, you will eventually be satiated sooner. Because it takes about 20 minutes until your brain registers that it's full, if you can focus on slowing down while you are eating you can reduce food intake.

Healthy Eating

Relying heavily on experts who tell you that their way is the only way to eat healthily can be dangerous. It can change from person to person in terms of what is healthy. But healthy eating in general does include recommendations such as don't eat out of a box too much and eat food in their natural state. Missing out on nutrients can create a starvation feeling in the body and can create resistance to weight loss because your body will hang on to fat. How about gluten? Listen to your body, and pay attention to symptoms such as gas or bloating to determine if it's okay for you to eat. I am originally from Europe, and gluten is just fine for most people there, even after they move to the United States. Gluten sensitivity is present in my life via bloating, but I am not willing to give up some of the yummy products that contain gluten for the rest of my life. I eat it occasionally, but I have no rule for how many times or what time of the day. The more relaxed I am around it, the less I want it.

Implement Daily Nutritional Commitments

While I was studying the hormonal impact of nutrition at Metabolic Effect, I learned more about blood sugar regulation in the body via food intake. Jill Coleman, MS, one of the owners of the company, taught me about implementing daily nutritional commitments. She said, "Nutritional commitments are high-impact, low-effort behaviors, and they are useful to create freedom around food. They help us feel more satisfied and satiated. Thus, we don't ever reach the point of needing to overindulge." It is not about doing everything perfectly but about creating a good baseline for how you want to care for yourself though nutrition. Therefore, keeping your blood sugar in check and preventing huge drops during the day is important for weight management, and it also helps prevent overeating patterns, as they help to limit feelings of deprivation.

Your nutritional commitments will be different than mine, but that is where you have to do the work toward maintaining stable blood sugar.

My nutritional commitments are as follows:

- When I get hungry, I start the day with a protein-based breakfast to feel satisfied and satiated.
- Eat a huge meal based on salad every day, at least once a day to prevent myself from having physically driven overeating or binging as a result of a lack of nutrients.
- Eat protein for at least two main meals in order to feel satisfied and satiated.

If I don't implement these regularly, I have a tendency to crave sweet drinks and sweet food all the time, as my blood sugar drops, and all I want is something sweet and quick to get back my energy.

What are your daily nutritional commitments? Consider making a list like mine.

Weight Management with Nutrition

There are countless diets telling you what to eat, but your nutrition plan is unique; you are the only one who can tell what's best for you. Let's discover your plan.

Energy Regulation

Normal eating requires you to understand what foods make you feel satiated for hours. This requires tuning in to your unique body and how it feels. Understanding the connection between carbohydrates, fats, proteins, and energy regulation will help you take charge of your blood sugar and eventually your energy. This helps you avoid all day long.

There are only three different kinds of macronutrients in foods: proteins, carbohydrates (carbs), and fat. The amount of each that you need to initiate fat loss, manage your weight, maintain energy, stave off hunger, and reduce cravings is different for everybody.

The tipping point of blood sugar regulation is when you have stable blood sugar in the form of mental and physical energy, but you can also successfully manage your weight. This is trial and error at first, and then it becomes automatic. Blood sugar regulation is the primary factor for fat loss and weight management.

Food provides both calories and information for the body. Protein, fats, and carbohydrates impact hormones differently. Normal eating allows you to address all these aspects of blood sugar regulation.

Creating hormonal balance in your body allows for the two of the most critical aspects of weight management, eating the right amount of calories and balancing insulin levels. Most of us want to eat less and less calories and thereby lower our insulin. This is a common mistake, even among professionals and fat-loss experts, where the mantra, "lower is better," is repeated all the time.

Let's take a closer look at carbs, protein, and fat to see how they regulate blood sugar.

Carbs that support energy regulation and stable blood sugar:

- Are nutrient-dense whole foods
- Are available in nature
- Can be metabolized at a cellular level by carrying easily digestible nutrients

Carbs that don't support energy regulation and stable blood sugar:

- Are empty nutrients, which hamper an appropriate metabolism
- Can cause digestive issues
- Are processed (factory-made)

Understanding the impact of empty nutrients for energy regulation is vital, as they ultimately determine the success of your weight-management efforts.

In order to nourish your cells, the food you eat must be broken down into its constituents. For example, the moment you eat carbs, the body breaks them down and turns them into sugar.

To metabolize the carbs (sugar) within food, the body uses up energy in the form of micronutrients (vitamins and minerals). To turn carbs into cellular energy, your body needs minerals such as chromium, iron, copper, magnesium, zinc, and vitamin B.

We all need energy from food to keep going. Your physical and mental energy is based on your cellular energy. When you consume either nutrient-dense food or foods that lack nutrients, you decide what kind of energy you create on the cellular level.

Nutrient-dense carbs like roots, tubers, vegetables, and fruits give your body an immediate nutritional deposit that it needs to turn calories from carbs into energy. Foods that lack nutrients, on the other hand, demand that your body releases micronutrients (vitamins and minerals), cofactors that help you use the calories you have just eaten.

Carbs are always an easily available fuel source for your cells. They are broken down into glucose (sugar) whether you eat a sweet potato, a piece of apple pie, or the apple itself. Carbohydrates are the most easily used energy source because of their rapid breakdown and their release into the bloodstream. They can quickly raise your blood sugar. In order for your body to keep your blood sugar in a healthy range, a hormone called insulin is secreted to help level out your blood sugar. The level of insulin in your body is highly influenced by the carbohydrates you eat.

Just like your car, your cells need fuel to function. Your body's easy source of fuel is sugar. When you eat, your body breaks down the food to digest it and to be used for fuel and nutrients. All carbohydrates, even healthy ones, turn to sugar in the body; all carbs therefore trigger the release of insulin, a powerful fat-storing hormone.

The more insulin you have in your bloodstream, the fewer carbs you can safely process. And the more sensitive to carbs you are, the greater the degree of insulin resistance. When your cells became more resistant to insulin, you became more sensitive to carbs. It is a vicious cycle.

Carbohydrates and insulin are buzzwords these days. Experts recommend people cut carbohydrates from their meals, and calories are cut to lose weight faster. This can only cause insatiable hunger, uncontrollable craving, and unbalanced energy in the long run. This ultimately creates a lack of energy, changes in mood, less and less energy for workouts, and loss of muscle is inevitable. Muscle is important for an optimum metabolism, and insulin must be produced to maintain muscle mass.

The Role of Insulin

Primary Function of Insulin

When a carbohydrate is digested and broken down in the body, glucose (sugar) enters the bloodstream. Whether you are eating bananas, apples, beans, rice, pasta, corn, or dried fruit the body turns them into sugar the moment you ingest them. After this, the pancreas secretes insulin into your bloodstream in response to dietary carbohydrates to do its primary function. Glucose, in fact, is the primary insulin release stimulator.

Insulin works like a messenger to help carbs (glucose) travel to the cells for energy use. In other words, it finds sugar and nutrients in your bloodstream and puts them where they belong, your cells.

Another job of insulin is to lower blood sugar, as high blood sugar is toxic. When you move to a new place and have to sort out where to put your stuff, what you need, and what you can throw away. Insulin does the same. It puts away the sugar your body can't handle to put your blood sugar levels back to normal.

Insulin sends a message to your liver and muscles to store any excess glucose as glycogen for later use. Therefore, insulin is a storage hormone.

When you eat carbs, your body checks in with your liver and your muscles to see how much stored sugar is there; based on the answer, it will decide what to do with the next carbs you ingest. If you have some free space, your body will refill it with the food you are eating.

Even though your body has limited amount of space to store carbs, it has unlimited space to store fat. So, when you eat more sugar than your body can store in your muscles or liver, the latter has nowhere to put the extra carbs, so it turns them into one of the two types of fat: triglycerides (circulating blood fat) or adipose tissue (body fat). In other words, if all your glycogen storage sites are full, and the excess sugar isn't used right away, the body converts the leftovers (glucose) to fat, a much longer-term fuel source that's far more difficult to burn off. There is only one exception to this rule: when you eat thirty minutes to two hours after exercising. Your muscles tap into the carbs to utilize sugar to be replenished and restored first.

If you constantly eat carbohydrates, causing your glucose level to be high all the time, insulin must work all the time to get the unnecessary glucose out of your bloodstream by turning it into fat. Basically, you put your body into fat-storage mode. By finding your carbohydrate tipping point, you lessen the amount of glucose being stored as fat,

Surprisingly, the body only needs about four grams of sugar in your bloodstream, equal to one teaspoon of sugar.

Does that mean eating more than one teaspoon of sugar is toxic? Not really. Your body's response to carbs largely depends on the type, the amount, and some other factors.

You need to become mindful of how much carbohydrates your particular body can handle so that only enough insulin is secreted to do its main job, helping the cells take in nutrients and storing some for later use. However, it's best not to have enough glucose in your body so that insulin is needed to store it as fat.

Don't push carbohydrates away in general just because, biochemically speaking, they are sugar and can get you in trouble when you store them as fat. They have vitamins, minerals, and fiber in them, all of which you need for energy and health.

I know it's easier when someone tells you exactly how much you should eat. But how is that working out for you so far? Only you know what's best for your body. What you can do is learn the basics and apply them to your life based on how you feel. Then you will not only have the perfect nutrition plan but also you will understand what you are doing. Isn't it refreshing to feel like an expert in your life?

These are the four main factors that influence how fast your blood sugar rises:

- The amount and type of carb in the meals you consume over time
- The amount of protein, fat, and soluble fiber in the same meal
- The frequency of your carb intake
- The body's individual ability to process them

Carbohydrates are information to your body, and the signals they send to your brain via hormones are what make you feel full or hungry. Therefore, the smart use of carbohydrates is one key to your weight management.

A low-carb diet is not necessarily better. The solution is rather to find the tipping point—the amount of carbohydrates that is low enough for fat loss or weight management but high enough to maintain energy, reduce cravings, and alleviate hunger.

In a nutshell, blood sugar imbalances can lead to weight management issues. High blood sugar creates blood sugar imbalances and high insulin production. Blood sugar imbalances make blood sugar drop, which creates hunger. Hunger leads to more frequent eating. More frequent eating prompts high insulin production. High insulin production activates fat-storage mode. Fat-storage mode means not burning fat for fuel.

Symptoms include:

- Blood sugar levels that rapidly rise or drop.
- Huge energy swings throughout the day. This can be a result of diets high in carbohydrates or refined foods.
- General fatigue.
- Blurred vision.
- Compulsive eating.
- Cravings for sugar and carbohydrates.

Too much insulin (after ingesting too many carbs) also causes you to consume more calories overall. According to Dr. Robert Lusting in the August 2006 edition of the journal *Nature Clinical Practice*

Endocrinology and Metabolism, insulin stimulates the appetite by working on the brain in two ways.

- Insulin blocks signals to the brain by interfering with the appetite-suppressing hormone leptin, causing you to eat more.
- Insulin causes a spike in dopamine, the hormone that signals the brain to seek rewards. Dopamine then spurs a desire to eat in order to achieve a pleasurable. No wonder putting down the fork is so tough. One of the primary effects of excess carb consumption includes a dopamine rush, the same mood hormone released with other addictive behaviors, such as out-of-control gambling, sex addiction, drug or alcohol abuse, or smoking. We can basically place carbs and sugars into the same category.

Cause of Insulin Overload

Here are some of the main culprits for excess insulin:

- Consuming too many nutrient-poor carbohydrates—the type found in processed food, sodas, and other sugary drinks—and foods containing high-fructose corn syrup, packaged low-fat foods, and artificial sweeteners,
- Consuming healthy carbs in excess amounts, such as beans, legumes, potatoes, grains, and high-carb fruits like pineapple, banana, and so forth.
- Insufficient protein intake.
- Inadequate fat intake.
- Deficient fiber consumption.
- Chronic stress.
- Lack of exercise.

Aside from the tasks of insulin previously described, it also absorbs and stores amino acids from the protein you eat to build muscle. Insulin is the key to feeding your cells. In other words, to create body change, you need enough insulin to build muscle but not enough to store fat. Rather than simply trying to lower insulin to extremely low levels and possibly losing muscle in the process, it is far better to maximize insulin sensitivity.

Therefore, the overall message insulin sends to the body is to build fat and muscle. Without insulin, you couldn't build muscle in the body, and you need your muscles to have an optimal metabolism.

Eating meals low in carbs and calories can give you a quick result in fat loss, but it also creates weight fluctuations because these plans are pretty unsustainable. Programs with this guideline rely heavily on willpower and make you constantly think about what food you can or can't eat.

The solution is to figure out what your body can handle and live accordingly. You don't have to blindly lower your calories or carbohydrates for quick results or live in constant fear of exceeding the limits. You actually know your body and can understand its tipping point in carbs, proteins, and fats and live accordingly. This allows you to have stable blood sugar and a successful plan for weight management.

Finding your carbohydrate tipping point is important not only for energy regulation but also for weight management. The higher the level of insulin in you bloodstream, the greater the amount of fat you will retain in your fat cells. This is why it's important to focus on insulin sensitivity instead of simply lowering the level.

Carbohydrate Tipping Point

The phrase "carbohydrate tipping point" comes from *The Metabolic Effect Diet*, written by Keoni Teta and Jade Teta. It's a great way to capture the amount of carbs that are too much or too little for weight management. This is based on individuality, need, and preferences. We are all unique and require a unique blend of macronutrients. It is necessary to become a detective because you can then see how much carbohydrates are too much for your body to process. The amount of carbs, fats, and protein you should eat together to initiate fat loss or manage your weight, maintain energy, calm hunger, and reduce cravings is different for everybody.

When it comes to determining sufficient carbohydrate intake from nutrient-dense carbs, I've used Mark Sisson's tool, The Primal Blueprint Carbohydrate Curve, for many years with great success for myself and clients of mine who are more prone to gaining weight by eating carbs. Carbohydrate intake is a pivotal factor in fat loss, and lifestyle factors need to be taken into account.

The following guidelines will work best for a lot of people on average. They are a good baseline to start with.

0 to 50 Grams of Carbohydrates per Day: Ketosis and Fat Burning

The body can convert fat to energy. By keeping your carbohydrate intake near fifty grams per day, you are going to enter ketosis. In my professional experience, I worked with people whose body loved to be in this state and had stable energy throughout the day, but others had low energy in the long run. It really depends on your unique biochemical makeup. This is the type of plan that a lot of diets recommend, and you do lose weight.

I don't recommend staying on this plan forever because of unnecessary deprivation of plant foods, but if you are an inactive person, it will help you lose weight. Now, can you turn it into a lifestyle? Remember, if you lose weight with a nutrition plan that you can't keep up in the long run, most likely you will gain the weight back. The solution might be implementing some type of exercise in your life so that your body could handle more carbs.

You would consume starchy carbs or sweet fruits one meal per day, and the rest of your carbs would be greens.

50 to 100 Grams of Carbohydrates per Day: The Sweet Spot for Weight Loss

Eating at this range, you can still minimize insulin production. This is great for most people managing their weight, because it helps them to not rely on exercise to stay lean and fit. If you hit a plateau with this amount of carbs, I recommend you switch between zero and fifty grams and fifty to one hundred grams of carbs per week. It is good for people who are not very active or participating in high-intensity interval exercises regularly.

To get this amount daily, it would equal two meals a day with starchy carbs or fruits; the rest of your carbs would be greens.

100 to 150 Grams of Carbohydrates per Day: The Sweet Spot for Maintenance

If you are at your ideal body weight and composition, you can try to maintain it with this amount of carbohydrates; you'll enjoy starchier carbs, sweeter fruits, and lots of greens.

If you are doing resistance strength-training activities or if you have a moderately active job or lifestyle, you are more likely to get away eating this amount of carbs. However, if you don't do short, high-intensity training or strength training, you might need to lower your carb intake.

This plan would include three meals per day with starchy carbs or fruits high in sugar; the rest of your carbs would be greens.

150 to 300 Grams of Carbohydrates per Day: The Steady Track to Weight Gain

Eating this amount of carbohydrates is a great example of understanding the difference between healthy eating versus eating for fat loss or weight management. Although the food pyramid recommends this amount of carbs per day, unsuccessful dieters end up here, due to their frequent intake of sugar and grain products (breads, pastas, cereals, rice), including whole grains, and due to infrequent exercise or movement. If you do some type of intense cardiovascular activity for more than an hour per day, you have a very active job, or you have a stressful life that is demanding both mentally and physically, you can get away with this amount of carbs.

300 or More Grams of Carbohydrates per Day: The Weight-Management Disaster for Most People

As you know, carbs turn to sugar in the body, and what you don't use up for energy is converted to stored fat. It is easy to eat this amount of carbs based on the food pyramid, and you are likely to become obese; it may make you prone to get type 2 diabetes.

Chronic dieters make the mistake of avoiding carbs or keeping their intake under fifty grams per day, and then when they can't keep up their willpower, they enter the crash or binge cycle of dieting.

For fat loss, I usually recommend starting with one hundred grams of carb intake for a day in total. This is a good baseline. From this point, you can increase or decrease your intake in relation to two criteria: fat-loss results and monitoring your hunger, energy, and cravings.

Carbohydrates 101

Starchy Veggies:

Starches are plants that store glucose as starch, which is sugar
Starchy veggies include pears, corn, beats, yams, white or sweet potatoes, and turnips. Bananas, spaghetti squash, rutabagas, beans, lentils, and peas are also starches.

Nonstarchy Veggies:

These are vegetables like broccoli, salad greens, cauliflower, cucumber, zucchini, spinach, peppers, onions, and many more.

It is important to understand that for your body, sugar is the same thing as starch. Biochemically speaking, they both turn to sugar and then to glucose.

Grains:

Rice, oat, barley, wheat, and flour-based products such as bread, pasta, cereal, and many more.

Fiber:

Soluble and insoluble fiber exists.

Soluble fiber:

- The kind found in fruits and veggies

Insoluble fiber:

- The type found in grains, fruit, veggies—in the skin, the woody parts, and the structure of plants

Understanding the Difference between Starchy and Nonstarchy Vegetables

Not all vegetables count as vegetables in terms of nutrition. Root vegetables don't count, for example. They are high in starch and include potatoes, sweet potatoes, squash, parsnips, and artichokes.

Don't worry about eating fewer calories; eat less starch if you want to lose significant amounts of body fat. This is one area overlooked in the diet industry. Check your diet to see if you eat a lot of starchy carbs as vegetables that are preventing you from losing or managing your weight.

The same goes for fruits. They are natural food products. If you are managing your weight, don't worry about avoiding them. But eating too much of anything sweet, even fruits, can cause higher levels of blood sugar, which limits fat burning.

Glucagon and Protein

Balancing blood sugar depends on more than getting the right amount and the right type of carbs. Nature, by default, offers some great nutrients for promoting healthy bodies and also helps balance blood sugar; in turn, this helps promote fat loss or weight management.

Fat-storage mode is induced by having a high insulin level, but fat-releasing mode is determined by having a high amount of glucagon in your body. Insulin and glucagon are counterregulatory hormones. This is because insulin's main job is to help store nutrients in your body, but glucagon's main job is to pull nutrients from their storage sites for fuel.

When insulin is present in the bloodstream, glucagon cannot do its job. On the other hand, when glucagon is prevalent in the bloodstream, it can signal fat and glucose to be released from storage for use as fuel.

You need protein to feel full for a long period of time and to have energy throughout the day. Protein is molecularly dense, and it doesn't produce nearly as much insulin as carbs do. Many people try to get the protein intake from beans, but beans require a huge insulin response from the body because of the carbohydrate content. Therefore, animal protein is better.

A Unique Fiber-Rich Diet Increases Satiety

Eating more fiber-based foods is the key to successful weight management. No expert would argue on this advice, but it is misunderstood. Understanding the fiber content of carbs relative to other ingredients is the key to successful weight management.

You hear all the time that grains, beans, and legumes have the highest fiber content, and that's why you should eat them. It is true that they have more fiber compared to fruits and veggies, but when it comes to weight management, this is not what matters.

As Dr. Jade Teta says, "for fat loss, you must consider the total sugar load relative to the fiber load. Fiber is important because it slows the release of glucose into the body and reduces the negative hormonal response. The problem is that the body still eventually has to deal with the total glucose amount in a piece of food, whether the fiber is present or not. It is better if it can deal with the glucose slowly, and fiber helps with this, but too much starch or sugar in general is not helpful for fat loss. So, if you really want to maximize fat loss and minimize fat storage, you should seek out carbohydrates that have the smallest amount of sugar or starch and the highest amount of fiber. Vegetables fit this description but grains do not. Consider processed white bread. This product is all starch with almost zero fiber. Compared to whole-grain bread, the fiber concentrations are clear. Now consider vegetables and fruits. They have less *total* fiber than whole grains but more *relative* fiber. This low starch-to-fiber ratio makes these foods better sources of fiber. Even beans, which are considered one of the highest sources of fiber, are two-thirds starch. That is not a great ratio as far as fat loss is concerned."

The best veggies, with the highest ratio of fiber to sugar, are kale, spinach, brussels sprouts, broccoli, green beans, collard, peppers, and leafy greens.

People need different amounts of protein or fat to have stable energy throughout the day. I recommend you tune in to your body and play around with the amount. This single tool of adding protein and fat to your meals or snacks can help you feel energized. Additionally, the recommended daily intake level of carbs only works with sufficient protein and healthy fats.

Following are recommendations for combining macronutrients:

- Start with eating twenty or thirty grams of protein with each main meal (about the size of the palm of your hand).
- Include two to four tablespoons oil or other fat daily (twenty-four to forty-eight grams); make sure they are naturally occurring, healthy fats.
- Add carbs based on your activity level and your sensitivity.

Healthy cooking fats include:

Plant-based fats: coconut oil and palm oil

Animal-based cooking fats: ghee, butter, lamb fat, duck fat, schmaltz (chicken fat), bacon grease, lard, or tallow (beef fat)

Healthy fats for cold use include:

- Macadamia oil
- Sesame oil
- Walnut oil
- Olive oil
- Nuts and seeds, including nuts and seed butters
- Flaxseed oil (for occasional use)

If you are vegetarian or vegan and have weight issues, consider what was just described about the consumption of carbohydrates.

Personally, I know many people who don't eat meat and still have great blood sugar and energy levels all day. They also don't have weight struggles. Their tipping point in carbohydrates is between 150and 200 grams per day, and by eating high-sugar fruits like banana, pineapple, and starchy carbs, they don't throw their energy up and down daily. They might be luckier than most of us, because the rate at which their body digests the carbs and the amount of insulin secreted somehow gives them steady energy for long hours after meals.

If you have weight issues and don't want to eat animal protein, another interesting fact is that fat consumption makes carbs far more detrimental in terms of fat storage. Fat and carbs together produce more insulin than eaten alone. If you are vegan or vegetarian, lowering your fat intake with your high-carb meals can actually decrease the negative influence carbs have on fat storage.

Monitor Your HEC (Hunger, Energy, and Cravings)

Part of normal eating is using your biofeedback tools to gain insight into how your body feels and what it needs. The biofeedback amounts of hunger, energy, and cravings (HEC) need to be balanced; otherwise, there is no way you can sustain any body change effort. HEC is your body's hormonal feedback mechanism, so pay close attention to it. The proper response should be no hunger between major meals, no physical signs of hunger, and increased energy. You should also feel motivated and focused without anxiety and depression. Gas and bloating should not be present, and sleep should normalize.

The phrase "tipping point" helps you discover your body's unique needs when it comes to carbs, protein, and fat. It refers to a feeling where your hunger, energy, and cravings (HEC) are balanced, and you feel good with stable energy throughout the day, as mentioned previously. The more stable energy (instead of food comas) you get from your main meals or snacks, the less you will think about food all day long, because you feel good and energized. This is a game changer, period.

Getting your tipping point correct for carbs, fats, and protein will balance your metabolic function. Get it wrong, and your body will let you know. Use the symptoms listed as follows to monitor the mix of energy you put in your body. Remember, no food works alone. Your intake of carbs, protein, and fat together needs to be regulated. By monitoring your HEC (hunger, energy, and cravings) between meals and days, you can observe your own hormonal balance.

Hunger: Hunger is a physical sensation you feel in your body. To make sure you work with your hunger, fill your plate with nutritious food, including proteins and healthy fats with carbs. This combination will have the greatest satiety factor (feeling of fullness).

Energy: Your energy level can vary after eating. Having balanced energy after each meal means you have found your tipping point where the amount of food eaten is balanced for your metabolism. You don't feel sluggish or sleepy. Instead, you have created a hormonal soup wherein your mind is clear, and you are able to focus and feel energized for hours after eating.

Cravings: Recognizing the difference between a craving and true hunger is an important distinction. I went into great details about cravings in a previous chapter. Hunger is physical, and cravings are mental and emotional. As your body and brain communicate via hormones and neurotransmitters all the time, they are constantly giving you signals about what's going on with you. Mental and emotional states are big part of cravings, but remember not to overidentify with your thoughts and feelings. You have them, but they are not necessarily true.

Your brain chemistry and the hormones in your body, including stress hormones, are very much a component of hunger, energy, and cravings. Instead of practicing black-and-white or all=or-nothing thinking, implement flexible thinking when you listen to your biofeedback tools to monitor and adjust your eating or lifestyle. What makes you feel full, energized, and free of cravings day after day depends on many factors, not just the food you eat. Some of these factors for stable energy include maintaining quality sleep, preventing overtraining, paying attention to what and how you eat for optimal digestion, and managing stress levels.

Tipping Point, Weight Management, and HEC

Your biofeedback measures need to be in check; otherwise, it will be difficult to sustain efforts to change your body. If your goal is to lose weight (fat), and your hunger, energy, and cravings are stable, you can be assured that things are balanced, but you will need to monitor your fat loss. If all the biofeedback sensations (HEC) are stable and you are losing fat, you have found your carbohydrate tipping point. All you need to do is stay there. Do not try to cut carbs further. Doing so will sacrifice your energy level and make your fat-loss results unsustainable.

If the biofeedback sensations are not stable, or if they are stable but you are not losing fat, you have not found the tipping point yet. You will need to alter your plan in one of two ways described in detail in the next paragraph.

When it comes to balancing HEC (hunger, energy, and cravings) and weight management, Dr. Jade Teta, the author of *Metabolic Effect Diet*, puts it in a simple and understandable way: If sensations (HEC) are not balanced, increase the amount of fiber, protein, and water you take in. This is important. More times than not, the issue has nothing to do with carbs but is actually a protein issue. Wait a few days. If you are still having issues, raise your protein and fiber content one more time. If this is still not effective, increase the starch content of your meals a little at a time until the issue is resolved. This is a trial-and-error phase, wherein you need to alter your intake of the major macronutrients to find your unique fat-loss formula. This takes time and patience for some. But once you find it, you have a system for body change that will never fail you, even when your metabolism changes as you age. If all hormonal sensations are stable and you are not losing fat, decrease the amount of starch you consume at each meal by five to ten grams. Also, begin to look at your fat and sodium intake. Adjust your fat, carbs, and sodium intake downward every few days until your fat comes off. As you do this, you should be ramping up your protein and vegetable intake. Often, this is the stage where you will learn the difference between healthy food and fat-loss food. If managing carbs and fat is not giving the desired results, look at fruit and dairy next. These are two sources of sugar that can keep many from the results they want.

Finding your own formula and figuring out your tipping point to successfully manage your weight is important in the long run. For fat loss, I recommended dropping your carb intake to one hundred grams total per day. This can be a good starting point while you are measuring fat-loss results and monitoring your HEC.

If consuming fifty to one hundred grams per day as recommended is much lower than you have been eating, don't cut carbs out suddenly. Deviating significantly from the way you usually eat will move you toward the diet-binge cycle. Lessen your carb intake at one meal per day for a week until you reach the amount you are aiming for.

Gluten

I commonly get asked if food with gluten is bad for weight management. We are all unique, and I invite you to listen to your body and answer this question by yourself. With that said, here are some guidelines for you to consider:

- Eliminate foods that are common dietary irritants, such as diary, grains, legumes, and processed and refined foods.
- Reintroduce one of the eliminated foods after a month at each meal and see what effect they have on your daily energy level, including mental clarity, skin irritation, mood, and digestive function.
- Watch for common GI distress: gas, bloating, constipation, or diarrhea.
- Every five days, reintroduce another eliminated food to see which one might be causing issues.

Gluten-containing foods, such as bread, pasta, and pizza are also called trigger foods by the diet industry, fitness professionals, and nutritionists. I used to be one of them. Now, I have a different opinion on the subject.

The more you forbid something—exactly what the dieting mind-set does to you—the more you are going to crave it. People of different shapes and sizes who are not concerned about weight issues are much less impacted by these so-called trigger foods because they are not afraid of them and hence don't restrict them. By allowing themselves to eat these foods, they don't want them all the time.

As I mentioned before, gluten might be bothersome for your body; eliminating it is very highly recommended if so.

Nutrition for Cravings

In addition to discussing blood sugar regulation as the starting point for stable energy all day long, I would like to recommend a couple of nutrition-related useful tips against sugar cravings.

Your psychological state has an impact on your cravings and patterns or emotional eating; there are biochemical factors as well. For example, the brain chemical dopamine floods the brain when you seek and find pleasure. Cortisol, the stress hormone, is also involved in cravings. Therefore, dopamine creates a desire, and cortisol initiates the feeling of anxiety or uneasiness that pushes you to take action and seek out something sweet to eat.

Without going into all the science regarding these tips, I recommend you try them to see how they work for you. I firmly believe that even if they work for many people, they might not work for you. That doesn't mean they are not good options; it means that for you, at this point in your life, not all of them are effective for you in particular. What works for you will greatly depend on your metabolism, your mental and emotional state, and your personal preferences.

- If you regularly have sugar cravings, make a homemade broth. It can give you minerals and amino acids that your body needs. It is not that you should drink broth when you have sugar cravings; rather, drink broth often to prevent these cravings.
- Mix one tablespoon of cocoa powder into hot water (pour water onto the cocoa slowly while stirring to avoid clumping). You can also add raw honey, molasses, or stevia as well as cinnamon,

cayenne, or other spices to taste. To get the benefits of cocoa, you should drink it alone, not mixed into foods, protein powders, or milk. This drink can decrease hunger and cravings. It increases dopamine and serotonin, the feel-good hormones. It also helps if you are eating few carbs or entering the luteal phase of your cycle.

- L-glutamine can also help with sugar cravings. Put a teaspoon of it in some water or right on your tongue.

Here are some additional tips:

- Don't replace real sugar with artificial sweetener because artificial sweetener not only causes long-term health damage but it can also stimulate your appetite and carbohydrate cravings.
- Say no to fat-free products
- There is no perfect diet out there. You don't find one; you create one.
- Improve your sleep habits. Lifestyle factors such as sleep and stress have no calories; you can't eat them, but they significantly impact how much you eat and what you choose.
- Calories matter in weight management, but the impact calories have on hormones matters more related to hunger, energy, and cravings.

Best Approach to Fat Loss through Nutrition

The calorie approach is based on old science. Achieving hormonal balance within the body gets results. Hormonal balance can be achieved through the following steps:

- Adequate sleep (this supports cortisol regulation, which is crucial for hormonal balance)
- Healthy digestive function
- Successful blood sugar regulation by eating the right amount of carbs, based on your activity level (fifty grams per day or less with sedentary lifestyle; fifty to one hundred grams per day with active lifestyle)

- Adding more protein to feel satiated for a longer period of time if you are often hungry
- Increasing healthy fat intake and lowering carb intake to regulate blood sugar
- Replacing depleted nutrients (processed foods) with nutrient-dense food

If all of this chapter's information is not backed up with an inner freedom and tuning in to how the body feels, calculating grams of anything will lead to obsessiveness. Understanding how food influences hormones, body weight, and energy regulation was the main purpose, but I strongly discourage counting and calculating food on a daily basis. Focusing on grams, calories, and food groups regarding what to eat can create compulsive behavior around eating. If you are still sucked into it, reread the chapter "Build a New Home in Your Body."

Part VI How to Transform Your Body through Exercise

Although health and fitness professionals rely on exercise when it comes to weight management, the type of issue you are struggling with is not based on whether you exercise regularly. Fitness is helpful, but you can only do so much with training. And I'm sure you see the proof of it. Since nutrition is the driver in fat loss or weight management, and exercise is the backseat driver, you need to take care of the diet-binge cycle or the emotional eating aspect of your weight fluctuation first.

Finding Joy in Exercise

Do you have to push yourself to exercise like you push yourself with diets? Do you avoid exercise? Unfortunately, we often associate exercise with good or bad, and that creates stress in most of us. Exercise used to represent a sacred relationship with our body, but the fitness industry has created an image in our heads that we need to get better and faster every day. This leads to disappointments, and we instead avoid exercise. When I hear people say, "I am too lazy to exercise," "I have no time to exercise," or "I am intimidated to work out," I know these statements are only the symptoms behind the real reason they don't exercise. Lack of self-care is one of these reasons, for sure, but the bottom line is that we don't feel worthy of taking care of our bodies. We don't want to face the internal struggle we have developed between our physical body and the innate desire to move our body because it feels good.

Exercise has been called the most effective weight-loss tool, and many times when people lose weight, they also lose the willingness to work out. So they stop exercising, thinking there is no more need for that. And the weight comes back again.

Until you think you are worthy of everything in life because you exist, it will be difficult to come from a place of appreciating your body. When you can treat yourself with respect, regardless what you have done or achieved in any given day, only then can you manifest a natural appetite for exercise. We are meant to move to shift our energy (emotions and feelings) inside of us, and the emotional benefit we get by moving our body is to experience our own true power. Overcoming years or even decades of weight struggle by using exercise for permanent weight loss can be a great tool. But this is the case only if you first relearn how worthy you are, no matter what. Instead of beating up your body by forcing yourself to exercise, a workout will be a natural response coming from your innate desire to take care of your physical body.

With that said, when it comes to burning fat and managing weight, we really need to get into the hormones rather than just talking about calories. You usually hear about people counting calories and how many they burned through exercising. But exercise is really about what kind of hormones you produce.

Focus on Hormonal Impact of Exercise Instead of Calories

Choose an exercise that turns on the hormonal fat-burning potential, and burn more fat calories during and after the workout.

The best way to burn fat and boost your energy is with high-intensity interval training (HIIT), a type of workout where you alternate between short bursts of movement with less intense periods of activity or complete rest. This style of training can be done with your own body weight, with free weights, or on the weight machines and other exercise tools. It is not about what tools you use during the exercise but the style of training.

Don't be intimated by the term "high-intensity," because that's different for everybody. You can do it at your own pace, customizing it to your body and fitness level.

I recommend this type of exercise because with long, steady-state cardio, you only burn calories while you train. With HIIT, you burn calories even while you are at rest. In other words, you create what's called excess post-exercise oxygen consumption (EPOC). You experience an oxygen deficit when you are out of breath because of the high-intensity training is an anaerobic exercise made up of brief, strength-based activities such as sprinting, weight lifting, or jumping. When your workout is over, your body keeps burning calories and fat cells, essentially catching up on the oxygen it lost.

There are lots of studies and significant evidence that high-intensity intervals work wonders for burning fat and increasing cardiovascular health. It is not only more effective than long steady-state cardio but takes less time. When you go into full speed and then rest, you can't exercise for more than thirty minutes, and you don't have to. Because of the anaerobic properties, you get more benefit from twenty or thirty minutes of HIIT than you would with over an hour of cardio. It is the most efficient workout you can do, in my experience. Space isn't really a factor, either. I've done high-intensity intervals in my living room.

Nutrition is the most important tool when it comes to weight management, and while you are still working on figuring out your diet and patterns of emotional eating, I recommend you start practicing these exercises if you feel like doing them. It is good for your overall health. What's interesting about high-intensity training is that it not only helps you stay physically fit but also helps your emotions bounce back by relieving tension, anger, anxiety, fear of unknown, and uncertainty.

Keep in mind these suggestions before you start your HIIT to understand how to do it properly without injuries. Additionally, too much HIIT can lead to overtraining (chronic fatigue).

If you are a beginner, I am sure you are excited and motivated to kick off your new training program. Please don't make the mistake of working too hard. Although high-intensity is tailored to your fitness level, endurance, or strength, it can be too much on your body if you are not careful. I suggest first using cardio machines (treadmill, elliptical machine, and bikes) for interval training. It is easy on the joints and unidirectional. If you start sprinting immediately, you put yourself at greater risk for injury. If you consider yourself advanced I recommend doing HIIT with body-weight exercise, and then when you really get the hang of it, you can add different tools like weights, suspension training, kettlebells, medicine balls, bars, and so on.

Following are a couple of examples for this type of exercise:

Cardio Machine:

You can use any type of cardio machine for this type of exercise. The goal is to do short, intense exercise for an interval of twenty to forty seconds and then rest about a minute and then do it again six to ten times.

Body-Weight Training:

If you are at the track, sprint a hundred meters straight and walk every curve. The sprint is the intense burst for a short period of time, and then the active rest takes place while you walk around the curve instead of standing still.

You can also do compound movements such as squats, lunges, and burpees. An example of this type of exercise: Do ten body-weight squat jumps and ten burpees as well as ten push-ups and then rest for thirty seconds. Do this for ten minutes. It would be difficult to write a personalized exercise routine that's ideal for the fitness level of everyone who reads this book. I provide these examples so that you get the idea of the type of training I recommend.

Training with Weights:

The difference between this type of training and mainstream body building is that you don't wait a minute or so between sets with HIIT. You choose four exercises like squat with shoulder press, jumping lunges, steady plank (for a minute), and bent-over dumbbell row. You do the four exercises with a weight that allows you to do twelve reps, and then you stop when you run out of breath. Rest as long as you need to and then return when you are ready. Keep going with the four exercises until you need to rest, but do them four times overall.

At the end of your training, I recommend at least twenty minutes of walking to make sure you burn all the fat in your bloodstream that will be used by your muscles.

Most women and girls tend to shy away from weight training since that's what body builders do. However, it shapes the physique, adds curves, and preserves muscle, which makes you lean and toned. When you only do cardio, you can lose muscle and fat at the same time; weight training assures you are losing fat instead of muscle.

Please keep in mind that the intensity you start with has to match your fitness level. Don't compare yourself to others. Listen to your body and start from there. Take breaks when you need to, and return to the exercise when you are ready. Your workout should be based on you and on doing what feels right for your body.

The time for long steady-state cardio for effective fat loss or weight management is over. If you want to save time and be more effective in your fat-loss journey, go for the high-intensity interval training. However, if for some reason you have to force yourself to do this type of exercise, then I don't recommend it. Using willpower and constantly pushing yourself to work out doesn't give you happiness. I want you to commit yourself to some type of exercise though, ones that you enjoy. I happen to enjoy HIIT very much, so I don't have to force it. I also have periods when I get bored of it for months, and I do something else during that time. Sometimes I do nothing. I don't believe in forcing any type of exercise. I instead recommend you search for exercises you enjoy and stick with them. You can only feed your soul with exercises that you do enjoy. When you are able to connect with your body via exercise you enjoy, you will respect your body more.

Nutrition and Training

If your goal is fat loss, here are a couple things to keep in mind:

Athletes eat carbs (sugar) in their pre-workout meal because they need the energy for their training. However, if your aim is fat loss, you don't necessarily have to eat a lot of carbs in your meal before working out. Remember about the connection between carbs (sugar) and insulin. A high amount of insulin in your body will prevent you from being able to access and release stored body fat for energy. And to burn fat, you have to be in fat-releasing mode instead of fat-storage mode.

Post-workout meals can also vary depending on your goal. If you want to build muscle, I recommend eating high-carb meals with protein and a small amount of fat. This puts the sugar into your bloodstream quickly so that insulin delivers it to your muscles and absorbs the protein as well as building your muscle. But if you are more focused on fat loss, you don't have to eat a lot of carbs. Have a meal with protein, a small amount of fat, and as many veggies as you want.

Fats are necessary for healthy body function. But after training, I recommend them in small amounts no matter what your goal is. Fats will slow down the absorption of anything you eat (protein and carbs), so you get less benefit for fat loss or weight management.

FINAL THOUGHTS

You Can't Be What You Can't See

I want you to believe that peace with food and with your body is possible. Imagine and believe that there is a way of living where food doesn't have power over you. You can be in a state of mind where body image insecurity and an obsession with food is no longer part of your life. You have to believe what you want is possible. There is endless proof that people get out of very bad circumstances by believing that it is possible. There is also proof that people are able to succeed against the odds. And the only difference between succeeding and failing is your belief. There is a reason for where you are at this point in your life. You might think it's because of the skills and the know-how you acquired over the years. Although these are important factors, believing in yourself is even more important. With certain skills and know-how, you can hit walls, but when you believe that what you want is possible no matter what, you create an infinite opportunity for the possible.

Beliefs are not set in stone. If they don't serve you, change them. You have the power. It is time to set your limiting beliefs free and choose different beliefs. People don't become successful because they don't have challenges; they became successful because they believe in success. They keep going and trying until they learn enough from their obstacles and failures that they are able to succeed. Believing in yourself is an attitude you develop over time. Hopefully this book has been a great way for you to see how limiting beliefs or the root cause of your limiting beliefs—the feeling that you're not enough—is making you stop reaching toward your goals. If you do not consciously choose your belief, it is easy to fall prey to limiting beliefs you acquired by default in many areas of your life.

One of the greatest gifts you can give yourself is to overcome a self-conditioning belief that you were either raised to accept or that you picked up from social and cultural programing. If it doesn't serve you for good, you have to let it go or leave it where it originated.

Think about it this way: The world is nothing more than the projection of your beliefs. If you believe that you are worthy of happiness, love, comfort, fulfillment, success, joy, and peace, you can get them. If you believe these things are your birthrights and not only for special people can have them, then you will get there. You are actually already there; you just need to bring out the belief in yourself. You can only create a life that you believe in. It is as simple as that. You can make the journey from "I don't believe I am good enough" to "I believe I am powerful" because your birthright is to choose your life and beliefs.

The belief that you can have peace with food and your body image is more important than the skills and know-how to get you there. If you belief in it, you will find the way. Love and belonging are core needs for all humans, and we can't attain emotional health without them. Love can only be cultivated if we let our most vulnerable and powerful self be seen. Emotional health grows out of self-love and self-acceptance; without it, we break, fall apart, hurt others, and numb our feelings.

We all want to fit in and belong. Fitting in often means you do whatever it takes to belong, and you put your self-worth on the line. If they don't like you, you will likely attack your personality and feel ashamed. If your goal is to belong but you stay true to yourself, you feel disappointed if it doesn't work out and you might be sad, but you don't put your self-worth on the line. Therefore, being true to yourself supports your emotional health. Mind chatter and negativity bias are part of the human experience. You are fearful because it is ingrained in you; humans evolved to feel this way. Don't put your self-worth on what your mind chatter tells you.

Getting into self-worth and self-love is possible. Feeling a deep sense of love and belonging doesn't just mean the capacity to love other people. It also means you believe that you are loveable. This requires making different choices in your life to embrace vulnerability. Showing up in your life requires vulnerability on your part. Regardless of your socialization patterns or how scared you are to look behind your beliefs and discover your emotions or feelings, the way out of chronic dieting and compulsive eating is to feel your emotions and share instead of hiding and numbing them.

There is no failure on the road of life. Bumps will come up, and the precious gift they offer you will get you where you want to go. Your plan might fail, but you can't, as your self-worth can't be taken away. Be curious and stay resilient. It will get you where you want to be. We have the ingrained belief that when we stray from our diet and eat what we are not supposed to, we have fallen off the wagon. What if there is no wagon to fall off? This is your life all the time; you can't turn it off by falling off of it. Every experience exists to teach you something. It is your choice to follow the signs offered to you. Don't look for perfectionism; look for progress. You are not a problem—there is nothing to be fixed. Your weight and body issues are just trying to get your attention so that you wake up to your true potential.

The turning point in eating is in the process of turning toward your beliefs and feelings. Welcome how you feel, accept it, and stay present with why you feel the way you do. The ability to become vulnerable and have the courage to release your feelings is the key to permanent weight loss. Additionally, be willing to question the beliefs and feelings you have. If you are willing to go there, you hold the key to being free from weight issues, yo-yo dieting, and struggles with insecurity and feeling powerless around food and in your life. If you are not blindsided by focusing on overcoming the diet-binge cycle or emotional eating itself but you instead understand what you are truly hungry for going forward, being peaceful and having a happy relationship with your body is possible. When you satisfy your true hunger, you are on your way to savoring food and live again.

Made in the USA
Lexington, KY
14 November 2014